Adults Natural Remedy for Joint Pain

Empowering Joint Health, Nature's Nutrition, Effective Relief, and Powerful Support for Pain-Free Living

MIA METCALFE

Copyright Page

© 2023 [MIA METCALFE]

For inquiry please contact us

miahealthandfitnesscoach@gmail.com

GAIN ACCESS TO MORE BOOKS FROM ME

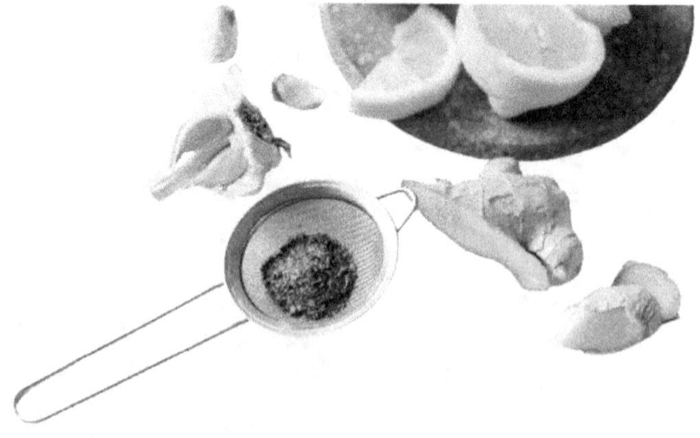

Table of Contents

Introduction

Lucy's life in the little village of Willowbrook was full of joy and adventure. Her tremendous vitality, however, began to diminish over time, replaced by the constant aching of joint discomfort. This unwanted companion threatened to rob her of her joy and vigor.

Lucy set out on a journey to locate a natural medicine that would provide relief from her agony, determined to recover her enthusiasm for life. She read books, spoke with experts, and combed the internet for answers. A ray of optimism arose from her studies.

Lucy's search led her to a treasure trove of natural cures, all of which promised healing and vigor. She meticulously crafted a regimen specific to her requirements, combining nature's healing power into her everyday routine.

Mornings started with a revitalizing cup of turmeric and ginger tea, its warm embrace healing her joints and energizing her soul. Lucy's kitchen was converted into a health-conscious haven, brimming with vivid fruits, veggies, and healthy grains.

Fatty fish, high in Omega-3 fatty acids, became a habit, and vibrant berries graced her breakfast, their anti-inflammatory characteristics a beacon of hope.

Lucy began on a journey of movement and awareness with the gentle instruction of a seasoned yoga instructor. Her haven became the class, where each stretch and posture whispered promises of strength and flexibility. Lucy's body responded with thankfulness as the weeks passed, her once-stiff joints giving to greater flexibility of action.

Lucy sought consolation in the embrace of nature during the peaceful afternoons, practicing deep breathing amidst the rustling leaves and singing birds. Meditation became her haven of quiet in the midst of the craziness of daily living. Lucy experienced a profound sense of inner calm as a result of this exercise, as well as a reduction in the intensity of her joint discomfort.

Lucy, who believes in holistic medicines, sought the help of a local acupuncturist and massage therapist. Their skillful touch untangles stress knots, providing comfort and relaxation.

Chiropractic therapy became an important part of her health regimen, helping to correct her spine and restore balance to her body.

Lucy created balms and compresses filled with natural treatments in her own home. Her tired joints felt immediate relief from the soothing touch of our homemade therapies. Hot and cold treatments, as well as Epsom salt baths, were beloved routines that provided relief at the end of each day.

Lucy's metamorphosis as the seasons changed was nothing short of remarkable. The previously restless soul now moved with elegance and ease, a tribute to nature's healing powers. Her laughter rang out across the community, a joyful symphony that touched everyone who knew her.

Lucy's trip showed her that with the correct knowledge and drive, even the most difficult problems could be conquered. Her tale became an inspiration, a ray of hope for people suffering from joint discomfort.

Lucy's story became legend in Willowbrook, a tribute to the remarkable power of natural treatments and a reminder that we all have the ability for healing and transformation inside us.

Understanding Joint Pain

Joint pain is a frequent complaint among adults, and it can have a substantial influence on everyday living. It happens when there is pain, stiffness, or inflammation in the joints, which are where bones connect and allow movement.

Adult Prevalence: Studies demonstrate that joint discomfort is common in adults, especially as they age. It is believed that more than 30% of individuals suffer from joint discomfort, with arthritis being the major cause. Arthritis alone affects millions of people globally, making it a major problem.

Types of Joint Pain: Joint pain can appear in a variety of forms, ranging from acute to chronic. Acute joint pain occurs suddenly and is frequently the consequence of an accident or trauma, whereas chronic joint pain lasts for a lengthy period of time, generally three months or more. Chronic joint pain is frequently connected with osteoarthritis, rheumatoid arthritis, and other inflammatory diseases.

Understanding the fundamental Causes of Joint Pain: Understanding the fundamental causes of joint pain is critical for successful therapy.

Arthritis (osteoarthritis, rheumatoid arthritis, gout), overuse or repeated strain, traumas (such as fractures or dislocations), and inflammatory disorders (such as lupus or fibromyalgia) are all common causes. Furthermore, lifestyle factors such as obesity, bad posture, and insufficient physical exercise can aggravate joint soreness.

Natural Remedies are Important: While medical therapies can be helpful in controlling joint pain, natural remedies provide a more comprehensive and frequently complimentary approach. Dietary adjustments, exercise regimens, herbal supplements, and lifestyle changes are all examples of natural therapies. These strategies seek to relieve pain, decrease inflammation, and enhance general joint health without the possible negative effects of pharmaceuticals.

We'll go further into the many aspects of joint health in "Understanding Joint Pain," looking at successful natural cures, lifestyle changes, and alternative therapies that empower people to take responsibility of their joint health. By treating the underlying causes of joint pain, we may pave the road for a more comfortable, active, and satisfying life.

Brief Explanation of Joint Pain

Joint pain, a common ailment, can frequently function as a quiet impediment to living a full and active life. It causes a variety of symptoms ranging from slight pain to acute, chronic aches, affecting the quality of daily activities. This book is a collective effort that aims to explain the route to healing and vitality for anyone dealing with joint discomfort.

Explanation of Joint Pain in Brief

Joint discomfort is caused by the complicated network of joints in our body. These are the locations where bones come together to allow movement. When these connections are strained, inflamed, or damaged, pain signals are sent, warning us to possible problems. Joint pain can be caused by a variety of causes such as age, trauma, autoimmune diseases, and lifestyle choices.

In adults, joint pain is more than just a physical feeling; it is a dynamic force that can have a substantial impact on everyday living. The incidence of joint soreness is significant, impacting millions of people globally. It cuts across age, gender, and regional lines, making it a universal issue that needs smart, collaborative solutions.

This book is a tribute to the power of communal wisdom and shared information. We hope to deliver practical insights, holistic methods, and evidence-based solutions to reduce joint discomfort and improve overall well-being through a collaborative effort. We go on a path to a life free of joint pain by combining our understanding of the human body with the incredible potential of natural treatments and technological therapies.

Let us be led by compassion, curiosity, and a common purpose to empowering folks to recover their energy and live life to the fullest as we start on this joint initiative.

Prevalence in Adults

Joint pain is an unexpected foe in the quest of a bright and active life. It presents in a variety of ways, ranging from slight discomfort to persistent, severe pains, and affects people of all ages and walks of life. This book is a collaborative effort, demonstrating the value of shared information in the pursuit of joint pain alleviation.

Adult Prevalence

The prevalence of joint discomfort in adults is an unavoidable fact. It has an influence on millions of people globally, regardless of demographics or geography. Natural wear and strain on our joints occurs as we age, which can be hastened by variables such as lifestyle, profession, and underlying medical disorders. Over 30% of individuals are thought to have some sort of joint pain, making it a common and frequently overlooked condition.

The experiences of persons suffering from joint pain vary, but they are always connected by a desire for alleviation and vitality. The genuine potential for collaborative solutions arises throughout this joint journey. We want to navigate the complicated environment of joint pain by uniting our expertise, experiences, and insights, delivering effective techniques that allow individuals to regain their mobility and quality of life.

This book is a monument to the power of teamwork, bringing together medical expertise, holistic techniques, and the shared experiences of people who have navigated the difficulties of joint pain. We go on a journey together toward a life free of discomfort, embracing a future of mobility, energy, and well-being.

Importance of Natural Remedies

Joint pain may be a tough thread in the fabric of health and well-being. It infiltrates the daily lives of countless people, spurring a search for effective and long-term remedies. This book takes you on a trip that connects with the deep potential of natural therapies for relieving joint pain and improving overall quality of life.

Natural Remedies' Importance

The importance of natural therapies in joint pain alleviation cannot be emphasized. The power of nature's offerings remains unrivaled in an era of modern medical treatments. Natural cures include a wide range of techniques, ranging from dietary changes and herbal supplements to mindful practices and physical therapy. These approaches have the potential to relieve pain, reduce inflammation, and restore balance without the risks associated with some pharmacological therapies.

Natural therapies also take a holistic approach, recognizing that good joint health is linked to total health. They act in concert with the body's natural processes to engage its underlying potential to repair and restore. Furthermore, they frequently enable people to take an active part in their own health journey, developing a feeling of agency and self-care.

This book is a salute to nature's wisdom, an investigation of the numerous and effective tools it gives for individuals seeking joint pain treatment. We go on a road that celebrates the human body's innate power to heal and grow via a handpicked array of cures, practices, and insights.

Let us proceed with the idea that the remedies to joint pain are as different and distinct as the people who experience it. We harness the power of natural treatments together, paving the way for a life full of energy, mobility, and the delight of unrestricted movement.

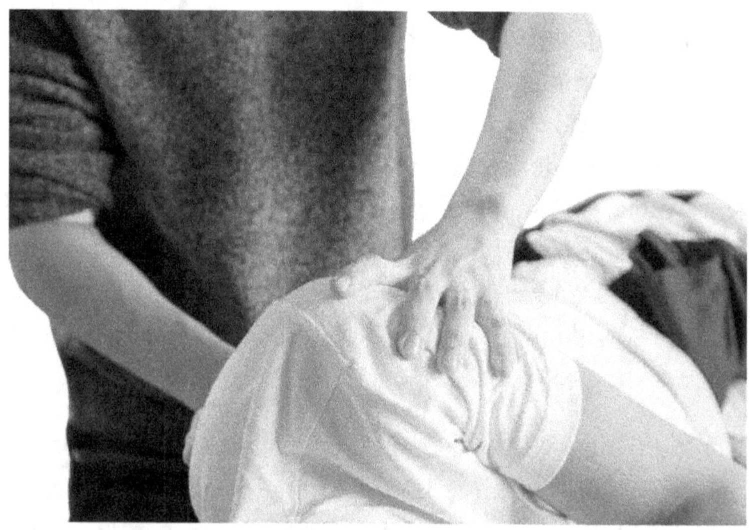

Chapter 1: Types and Causes of Joint Pain

1.1 Acute vs. Chronic Joint Pain

Joint pain is a complicated and multi-faceted ailment that can present in a variety of ways, each with its own distinct set of symptoms and underlying reasons. Understanding the distinctions between these terms is critical for proper management and therapy.

Acute Joint Pain vs. Chronic Joint Pain

1. Acute Joint Pain: Acute joint pain is distinguished by its quick onset and usually brief duration. It is caused by a single occurrence or injury, such as a sprain, strain, or joint damage. Pain is frequently severe, strong, and limited to the afflicted area.

- Accidents, sports injuries, and rapid movements that place undue stress on the joint are all common causes of acute joint discomfort. It can also be caused by medical disorders such as bursitis, a condition in which the bursae (small sacs of fluid that cushion joints) become inflamed.

- Acute joint pain serves as a warning signal to the body, alerting it to impending damage or harm. It is a transient condition that usually improves with rest, ice, compression, and elevation (RICE) procedures and proper medical care.

2. Chronic Joint Pain: - Chronic joint pain, on the other hand, lasts for a long time, usually three months or more. It is not caused by a single occurrence or injury, but rather by chronic discomfort that can have a substantial influence on everyday living.

- This sort of pain is frequently linked to underlying medical diseases such osteoarthritis, rheumatoid arthritis, and other autoimmune illnesses. In many circumstances, joint pain is caused by persistent inflammation, cartilage wear and tear, or an excessive immune response directed at the joints.

- Obesity, sedentary activity, and poor posture are all factors that might contribute to chronic joint pain. These practices can lead to joint strain and an increased sensitivity to persistent pain over time.

Joint Pain Causes

1. Arthritis - Arthritis, which includes osteoarthritis, rheumatoid arthritis, and gout, is a primary cause of joint discomfort. Osteoarthritis is caused by the slow disintegration of cartilage, which causes bone-on-bone contact and discomfort. Rheumatoid arthritis is an autoimmune disease in which the body's immune system assaults the joints by mistake, producing inflammation and discomfort. Gout, on the other hand, is caused by the buildup of uric acid crystals in the joints, resulting in extreme discomfort.

2. Overuse and repeated Strain: Continuous and repeated motions, which are widespread in particular vocations or hobbies, can contribute to joint overuse. This can cause tension and, eventually, joint discomfort. Overuse is frequently the cause of conditions such as tendinitis and carpal tunnel syndrome.

3. Injuries: Injuries including fractures, dislocations, or ligament tears can cause acute joint pain. The damage impairs the joint's natural functioning, causing pain, swelling, and reduced movement until the injury heals.

4.Inflammatory Conditions: Lupus, fibromyalgia, and psoriatic arthritis are all conditions characterized by persistent inflammation in the body, which can cause joint pain as a prominent symptom.

Obesity, bad posture, and a lack of regular physical activity can all contribute to joint discomfort over time. Excess weight puts additional strain on weight-bearing joints, while poor posture and inactivity can cause muscle imbalances and joint pain.

Understanding the differences between acute and chronic joint pain as well as the numerous underlying causes lays the groundwork for successful management and treatment options. Individuals can begin on a targeted strategy to alleviation and improved joint health by treating the exact kind and source of joint pain.

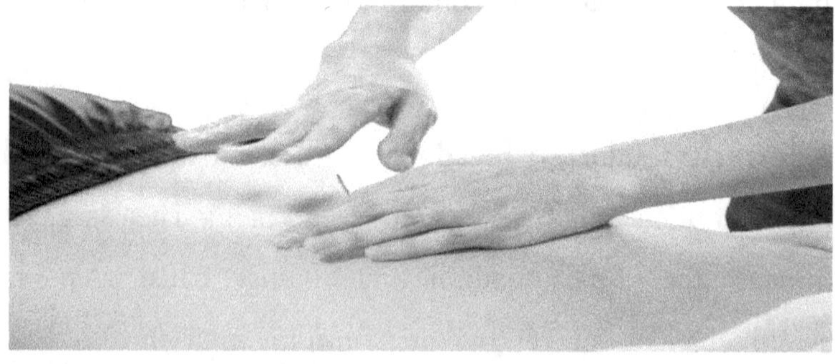

1.2. Common Causes (Arthritis, Overuse, Injuries)

Joint pain is a complicated phenomenon with several underlying causes. Understanding the underlying reasons is necessary for effective management and therapy.

Common Joint Pain Causes

1. Arthritis - One of the most common causes of joint discomfort is arthritis. It refers to a group of disorders characterized by joint inflammation. The two most prevalent varieties are as follows:

- **Osteoarthritis (OA):** This type of arthritis is caused by the slow disintegration of cartilage, which is the protective tissue that cushions the ends of bones. As cartilage deteriorates, bones may rub against one other, causing discomfort, stiffness, and decreased mobility, especially in weight-bearing joints such as the knees, hips, and spine.

- **Rheumatoid Arthritis (RA):** RA is an autoimmune disease in which the body's immune system assaults the joints, producing inflammation. This causes discomfort, swelling, and probable deformity in several joints, frequently symmetrically.

2. Overuse and Repetitive Strain: Continuous and repetitive motions, especially in certain vocations or hobbies, can contribute to joint overuse. This can cause tension and, eventually, joint discomfort.

Overuse causes conditions such as tendinitis (tendon inflammation) and carpal tunnel syndrome (pressure on the median nerve in the wrist).

3. Injuries: Traumatic injuries such fractures, dislocations, ligament tears, or sprains can result in acute joint discomfort. These occurrences interrupt the joint's regular functioning, causing instant discomfort, swelling, and generally restricted movement. Post-injury joint discomfort might last until the afflicted tissues recover completely.

4. Gout: - Gout is a kind of arthritis characterized by uric acid crystal accumulation in the joints. These sharp crystals can cause considerable joint discomfort, most typically in the big toe. Gout is impacted by heredity and is connected to dietary variables.

5. Bursitis: Bursitis is an inflammation of the tiny sacs of fluid (bursae) that cushion and lubricate joints. This might happen as a result of repeated motion, direct damage, or underlying disorders such as arthritis.

6. Lupus: Lupus is an autoimmune illness that can affect many regions of the body, including the joints. Lupus-related joint pain is frequently caused by inflammation, and it may be accompanied by other symptoms such as tiredness and skin rashes.

7. Fibromyalgia - Fibromyalgia is a chronic pain syndrome that affects the entire body, including the joints. It is thought to be linked to how the brain handles pain signals. Fibromyalgia patients may notice painful spots around joints.

Understanding the most prevalent causes of joint pain lays the groundwork for individuals to determine the underlying reasons of their suffering. Individuals might begin on individualized ways to alleviation and improved joint health by identifying the precise problem.

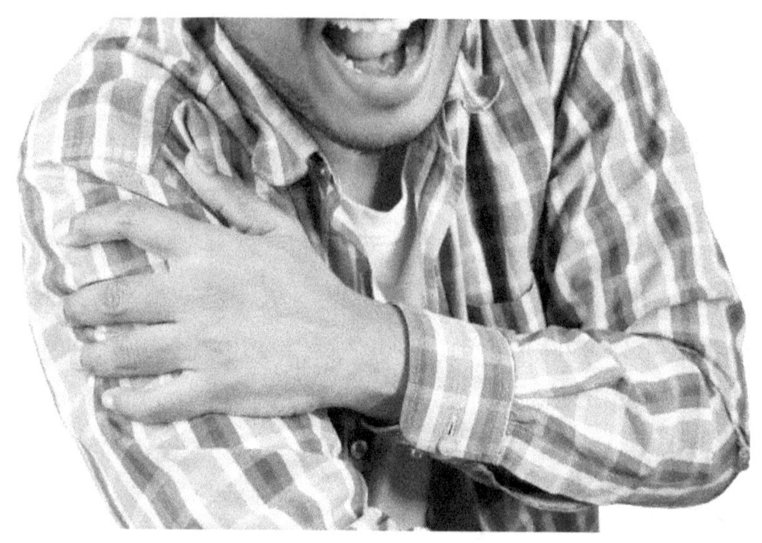

Chapter 2: Diet and Nutrition for Joint Health

2.1. Importance of Balanced Diet

Diet and nutrition are important factors in the health and function of our joints. A well-balanced diet not only supplies important nutrients for joint maintenance, but it also aids in inflammation management, tissue healing, and weight management.

The Importance of a Well-balanced Diet

1. Necessary Nutrients: A well-balanced diet contains a variety of vital nutrients that are needed for joint health. Vitamins (such as C, D, and E), minerals (such as calcium, magnesium, and zinc), and omega-3 fatty acids are examples. These nutrients help to create and repair cartilage, bones, and connective tissues.

2. Management of Inflammation: Chronic inflammation can aggravate joint discomfort and lead to diseases such as arthritis. Inflammation can be managed with a well-balanced diet rich in anti-inflammatory foods.

This involves including omega-3 fatty acid sources (such as salmon, walnuts, and flaxseeds) as well as antioxidant-rich foods (such as berries, leafy greens, and nuts).

3. Body Weight Management: Maintaining a healthy weight is critical for joint health, particularly in weight-bearing joints such as the knees and hips. A well-balanced diet aids in calorie control and supports a healthy body weight. It decreases joint stress, minimizing the likelihood of joint discomfort and illnesses such as osteoarthritis.

4. Bone Health: Having strong bones is important for joint stability and function. A healthy diet rich in calcium-rich foods (such as dairy products, leafy greens, and fortified meals) promotes bone health and lowers the incidence of fractures and joint problems.

5. Production of Collagen: Collagen is a protein that gives joints, tendons, ligaments, and skin structure. A healthy diet rich in protein (lean meats, poultry, fish, and legumes) supplies the building blocks for collagen formation, boosting joint strength and flexibility.

6. Hydration: Although it is sometimes forgotten, proper hydration is critical for joint health. Water lubricates joints, allowing for smooth movement. Dehydration can cause decreased joint lubrication, which can cause soreness and stiffness.

7. Preserving pH Balance: Some meals can alter the pH levels of the body, thereby affecting joint health. A well-balanced diet rich in alkaline-rich foods (such as fruits, vegetables, and some nuts) aids in the maintenance of an ideal pH balance, which supports joint function.

8. Restricting Trigger Foods: Certain diets, particularly those heavy in refined sugars, saturated fats, and processed carbs, can cause inflammation and joint pain. A healthy diet includes limiting these trigger foods.

9. Individually Tailored Approach: Individual dietary demands may differ depending on factors such as age, exercise level, and unique joint issues. Consultation with a healthcare practitioner or qualified dietitian can assist in tailoring dietary suggestions to specific requirements.

Individuals may make educated food choices that contribute to the well-being and longevity of their joints by knowing the critical role of a balanced diet in joint health.

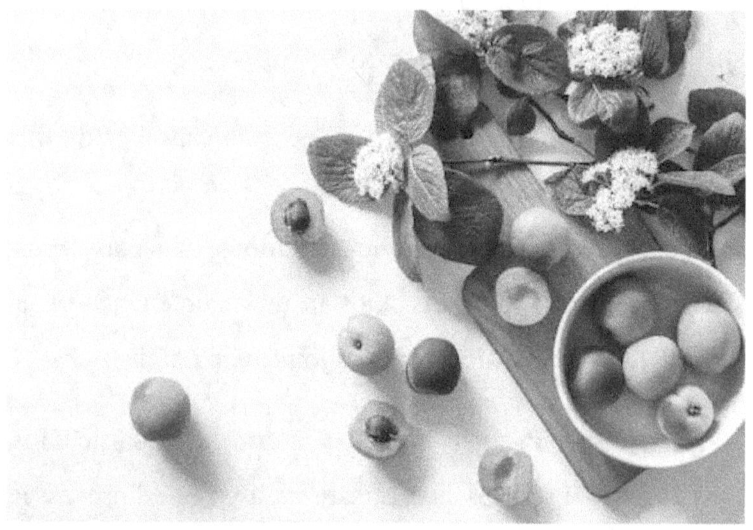

2.2   Anti-Inflammatory   Foods (e.g., fatty fish, turmeric, berries)

Adopting a diet rich in nutrients that promote joint health and help reduce inflammation is an important element of controlling joint discomfort. Incorporating anti-inflammatory foods into one's diet can be a highly effective natural treatment for joint pain.

Foods with Anti-Inflammatory Properties for Joint Health

1. Fatty Fish (Salmon, Mackerel, Sardines, etc.) Fatty fish are high in omega-3 fatty acids, which have anti-inflammatory qualities. These fatty acids aid in the reduction of joint inflammation, potentially relieving pain and stiffness. Regular ingestion of fatty fish can considerably improve joint health.

2. Turmeric: Turmeric is a golden spice recognized for its main ingredient, curcumin. Curcumin is a natural anti-inflammatory substance that aids in the suppression of inflammatory molecule synthesis in the body. It might be a beneficial addition to the diet for people suffering from joint discomfort.

3. Berries (such as blueberries and strawberries): Berries contain a lot of antioxidants, including flavonoids and anthocyanins. These chemicals have anti-inflammatory properties and aid in the protection of cells from free radical damage. Consuming a variety of berries gives an effective anti-inflammatory defense.

4. Leafy Greens (such as Spinach and Kale): Leafy greens are high in vitamins, minerals, and antioxidants, all of which benefit joint health.

They are high in calcium, which promotes bone health, as well as vitamin K, which aids in inflammation reduction.

5. Nuts and seeds (such as walnuts and chia seeds): Nuts and seeds are high in omega-3 fatty acids, making them a good option for people who don't eat fatty fish on a regular basis. They also include important minerals such as magnesium, which helps with muscle and nerve function.

6. Ginger: Ginger is yet another anti-inflammatory spice. It includes chemicals that have been demonstrated to relieve pain and inflammation, such as gingerol. Incorporating ginger into meals or drinking ginger tea might be good to joint health.

7. Green Tea: Green tea contains polyphenols, which are antioxidants with anti-inflammatory effects. Green tea can help fight inflammation and boost general well-being when consumed on a regular basis.

8. Olive Oil: Extra virgin olive oil is a staple of the Mediterranean diet and is known for its anti-inflammatory properties. It includes oleocanthal, a chemical having anti-inflammatory properties comparable to ibuprofen. Cooking using olive oil as the major source of fat can benefit joint health.

9. Pineapple: Pineapple includes bromelain, an enzyme that has anti-inflammatory qualities. Bromelain can help reduce inflammation and swelling, which may provide comfort for people suffering from joint pain.

Incorporating these anti-inflammatory items into one's diet can help substantially with joint pain management. To promote overall joint health, it's crucial to take a balanced approach, mixing these meals with a range of nutrient-dense choices.

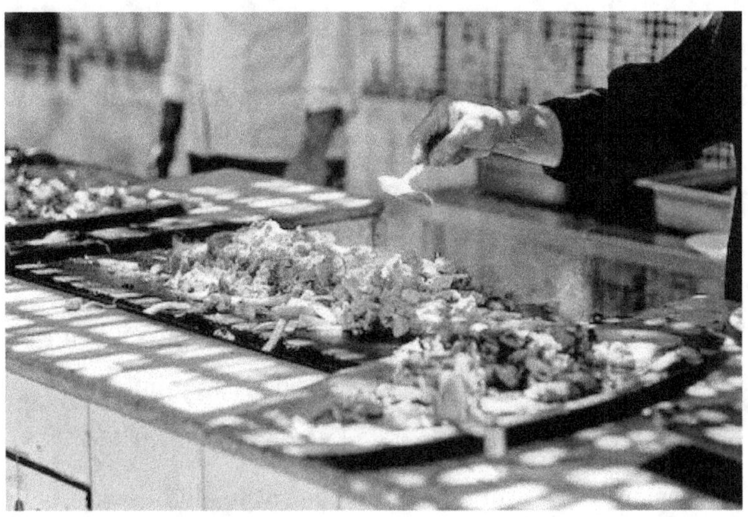

2.3 Role of Supplements (Omega-3, Glucosamine, Chondroitin)

While a healthy diet is the basis of joint health, some supplements can provide specific assistance to help with joint pain and inflammation control.

The Role of Joint Supplements

1. Omega-3 Fatty Acids: Omega-3 fatty acids, which are found predominantly in fatty fish such as salmon, mackerel, and sardines, are well known for their anti-inflammatory qualities. These essential fatty acids serve an important function in lowering inflammation in the body, making them an excellent supplement for anyone suffering from joint discomfort. Fish oil capsules, for example, can give a concentrated amount of these healthy fats.

2. Glucosamine: - Glucosamine is a naturally occurring chemical present in the body, specifically in joint fluid. It is essential for the formation and maintenance of cartilage. Glucosamine is a supplement made from shellfish shells. It is thought to help decrease cartilage deterioration and may improve joint pain and stiffness, especially in those with osteoarthritis.

3. Chondroitin: Chondroitin sulfate is a naturally occurring chemical present in cartilage and connective tissues. It is used as a supplement to support joint health, similar to glucosamine. Chondroitin is thought to help cartilage retain water, boosting its shock-absorbing qualities. It may also inhibit cartilage-degrading enzymes.

Synergistic Advantages

- Omega-3 fatty acids, glucosamine, and chondroitin frequently act together to enhance joint health. Omega-3 fatty acids help to reduce inflammation, while glucosamine and chondroitin are building blocks for cartilage repair and maintenance. When combined, they have the ability to provide full support for joint function and motion.

Dosage and Precautions: - Before beginning any supplement program, it is critical to contact with a healthcare expert. They may advise on proper dosages and make sure there are no interactions with other drugs or medical problems. Furthermore, obtaining supplements from reputed suppliers is critical to ensuring purity and efficacy.

Natural Food Resources: While supplements might be advantageous, several of these nutrients can also be gained via natural dietary sources. Consuming fatty fish gives omega-3s, while some shellfish can deliver glucosamine. However, attaining therapeutic levels purely through diet might be difficult, which is why supplements may be beneficial.

Complementary Approach: - Supplements should be used to supplement a varied diet rich in nutrients. They are not intended to replace complete foods, but they can give focused support for joint health, particularly for people suffering from disorders such as osteoarthritis.

Individuals may make educated judgments about including supplements like omega-3 fatty acids, glucosamine, and chondroitin into their joint health regimen by knowing the role of these aids.

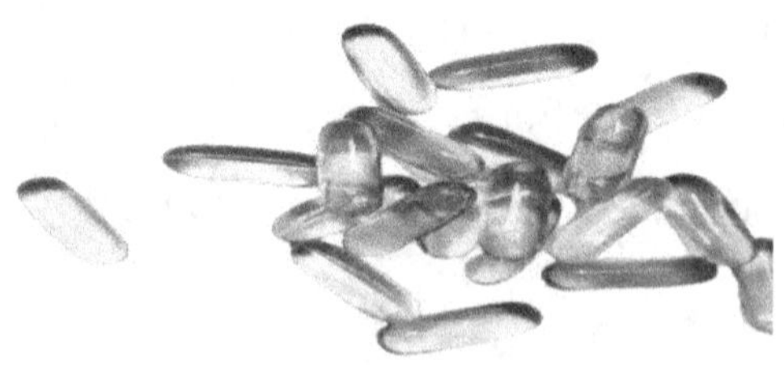

Chapter 3: Herbal Remedies and Supplements

3.1 Introduction to Natural Supplements

Natural supplements and herbal therapies have grown in favor as efficient pain relievers. They include a variety of chemicals that can help with inflammation, cartilage health, and general joint function.

An Overview of Natural Supplements

1. Zingiber officinale (Ginger) - Ginger is a multipurpose plant that contains potent anti-inflammatory effects. Its active ingredients, including as gingerols and shogaols, can help alleviate joint discomfort and swelling. Ginger pills, which come in capsules or extracts, are a popular alternative for people looking for natural treatment from joint pain.

Boswellia serrata (Boswellia serrata): Boswellia, often known as Indian frankincense, is obtained from the resin of specific plants. It has anti-inflammatory qualities due to the presence of boswellic acids.

Boswellia pills are thought to aid with joint discomfort, making them an important addition to the natural remedy arsenal.

3. Harpagophytum procumbens (Devil's Claw): The plant Devil's claw is endemic to southern Africa. Its roots contain iridoid glycosides, which are anti-inflammatory. Supplements containing devil's claw are often used to treat joint pain, particularly in disorders such as osteoarthritis.

4. Turmeric (Curcuma longa): Turmeric is a colorful spice rich in curcumin, a powerful anti-inflammatory ingredient. Curcumin has been widely researched for its ability to alleviate joint pain and inflammation. Turmeric supplements, which come in the form of capsules or extracts, provide a concentrated amount of this beneficial component.

5. Willow Bark (Salix spp.): Willow bark, obtained from willow tree bark, includes salicin, a natural chemical similar to aspirin. It has analgesic and anti-inflammatory effects. Individuals suffering from joint pain may benefit from taking willow bark supplements.

6. Stinging Nettle (Urtica dioica): Stinging nettle is a nutrient-rich herb that includes anti-inflammatory flavonoids. Individuals wanting to alleviate joint pain and inflammation may benefit from nettle supplements.

7. Glucosamine and Chondroitin Sulfate: Natural chemicals present in cartilage include glucosamine and chondroitin. They are available as a supplement and are thought to benefit cartilage health. These supplements may provide assistance for those suffering from osteoarthritis by improving joint function and reducing pain.

8.Consultation and Security: - It is critical to consult a healthcare practitioner or herbalist before adopting any herbal therapies or supplements. They may advise on proper doses, potential prescription interactions, and assure safety, particularly for patients with underlying health concerns.

9.A Holistic Approach: Herbal medicines and supplements work best when combined with a comprehensive strategy that includes a healthy diet, regular exercise, and other lifestyle changes. They provide targeted joint health support and can be useful components of a complete joint pain management regimen.

Understanding the possible advantages and concerns of herbal medicines and supplements empowers consumers to make informed decisions about including these natural aids into their joint health regimen.

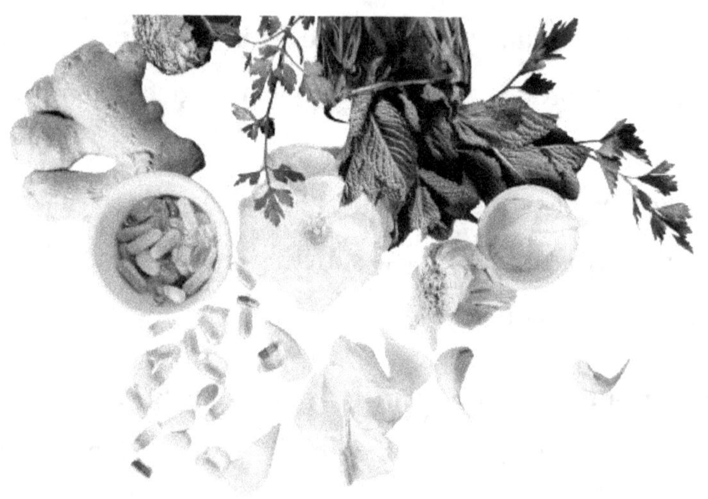

3.2 Benefits and Dosage Recommendations

Herbal medicines and supplements have gained popularity for their ability to relieve joint pain and improve overall joint health. Understanding their advantages and appropriate doses is critical for maximizing their natural joint pain reduction potential.

The Advantages of Herbal Remedies and Supplements

1. Ginger (Zingiber officinale)

Benefits: Ginger has anti-inflammatory characteristics, making it a useful natural cure for joint discomfort and swelling. It may also aid in the improvement of mobility and general joint function.

Dose Recommendations: For joint pain alleviation, a dose of 250-500 mg of ginger extract, taken up to four times day, is regarded safe and effective.

2. Boswellia (Boswellia serrata):

Benefits: Boswellia includes boswellic acids, which are anti-inflammatory. This makes it useful for those suffering from osteoarthritis and rheumatoid arthritis, since it may relieve pain and improve joint function.

Dosage Guidelines: A common dose of boswellia extract is 300-500 mg three times each day. It is critical to select a supplement that is standardized to contain at least 30% boswellic acids.

3. Devil's Claw (Harpagophytum procumbens)

Benefits: Devil's claw has anti-inflammatory and analgesic properties. It may help with joint discomfort, especially if you have osteoarthritis or another inflammatory joint condition.

Dosage Guidelines: A normal dose of devil's claw root is 2,500-3,000 mg per day, split into two or three doses. Look for a standardized extract that has 50-100 mg of the active ingredient harpagoside.

4. Turmeric (Curcuma longa)

Benefits: Curcumin, turmeric's active component, is a powerful anti-inflammatory agent. It can assist to alleviate joint pain and stiffness while also improving total joint mobility.

Dosage Guidelines: A normal dose of curcumin extract is 500-2,000 milligrams per day, taken with meals for better absorption. To improve absorption, look for supplements that include piperine (found in black pepper).

5. Willow Bark (Salix spp.): - *properties*: The salicin component of willow bark provides natural pain relief and anti-inflammatory properties. It may be useful in alleviating joint pain, making it a viable option to over-the-counter pain killers.

Dosage Guidelines: A typical daily dose of salicin is 240-480 mg, which is comparable to around 1-2 grams of willow bark.

Benefits: Stinging nettle contains chemicals that may decrease inflammation, perhaps providing relief from joint discomfort and swelling.

Dosage Guidelines: A common dose of stinging nettle root extract is 600-900 mg three times per day.

6.Glucosamine and Chondroitin Sulfate

Benefits: These naturally occurring substances promote cartilage health and may aid in the reduction of joint discomfort and mobility, especially in instances of osteoarthritis.

Dosage Recommendations: The typical dosage is 1,500 mg of glucosamine sulfate and 1,200 mg of chondroitin sulfate per day, split.

Considerations: - Before beginning any herbal remedy or supplement program, it is critical to see a healthcare practitioner, especially if you have underlying health concerns or are using drugs. They may make individualized suggestions while still ensuring safety.

3.3 Potential Interactions

While herbal medicines and supplements provide natural joint pain relief, it is critical to be mindful of potential interactions with drugs and other health concerns. Understanding these interactions ensures that they are used safely and effectively.

1. Zingiber officinale (Ginger)

Potential Interactions: Ginger may interact with blood thinners like warfarin or aspirin. It can increase the risk of bleeding by amplifying their effects. Furthermore, ginger may reduce blood sugar levels, therefore people who use diabetic medicines should keep a careful eye on their blood sugar levels.

2. Boswellia (Boswellia serrata)

Potential Interactions: Because it has comparable qualities to anti-inflammatory drugs, Boswellia may interact with them. Combining them may raise the chance of adverse effects. Before using Boswellia with prescription anti-inflammatory medications, check with your doctor.

3. Harpagophytum procumbens (Devil's Claw)

Potential Interactions: Similar to ginger, devil's claw may interact with blood-thinning medicines. When used with certain medications, it may increase the risk of bleeding.

Before any surgical treatments, it is critical to tell healthcare personnel about the usage of devil's claw.

4. Curcuma longa (Turmeric)

Potential Interactions: Turmeric may interact with blood thinners and antiplatelet medicines. It may increase the likelihood of bleeding. Turmeric may also interact with medications that lower stomach acid, thereby impairing their absorption.

5. Salix spp. (Willow Bark)

Potential Interactions: Salicin, which is similar to aspirin, is found in willow bark. When used with aspirin or other blood-thinning drugs, it may increase the risk of bleeding. Before taking willow bark in conjunction with these medications, ask your doctor.

6.Urtica dioica (Stinging Nettle):

Potential Interactions: Stinging nettle may interact with blood pressure drugs, perhaps causing blood pressure to drop even more.

It can also have an effect on blood sugar levels, thus diabetics should regularly check their blood sugar levels.

7.Glucosamine and Chondroitin: Glucosamine, like ginger and devil's claw, may interact with blood-thinning medicines. Chondroitin may also have minor interactions with blood thinners. Before any surgical operations, it is critical to tell healthcare practitioners about the usage of these supplements.

Consultation and interaction: Individuals must notify their healthcare physician about any herbal therapies or supplements they are using. Because of this open communication, possible interactions may be detected and controlled correctly.

Individualized Approach: Personalized counsel may be provided by healthcare practitioners based on an individual's unique health condition, drugs, and potential interactions. This assures that herbal therapies and supplements for joint pain alleviation are safe and effective.

Individuals may take a proactive approach to their health and make educated decisions about including herbal treatments

and supplements into their joint pain management regimen
by recognizing potential interactions.

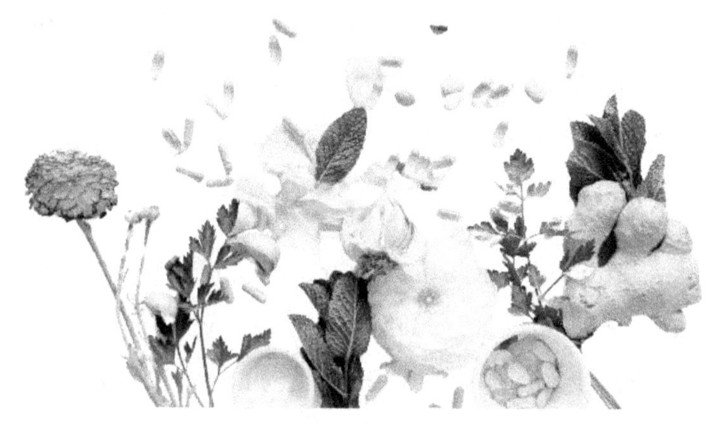

Chapter 4: Exercise and Physical Activity

4.1 Significance of Regular Exercise

Regular exercise is a cornerstone of joint health, providing a plethora of advantages for anyone looking for natural joint pain treatment. Understanding the importance of include exercise in one's daily routine is critical for preserving mobility and lowering pain.

The Importance of Regular Exercise

1. Strengthening Muscles and Supporting Joints: Regular exercise helps to strengthen the muscles that surround the joints. This additional support lessens the strain on the joints, reducing discomfort and improving general joint function.

2. Maintaining Joint Flexibility: Physical exercise promotes complete joint range of motion. This promotes flexibility and avoids stiffness, which is especially good for people suffering from illnesses such as osteoarthritis.

3. Promoting Cartilage Health: - Exercise helps to distribute synovial fluid, which nourishes and lubricates the cartilage that surrounds the joints. This mechanism promotes cartilage health while potentially decreasing degenerative processes.

4. Weight Management: It is critical for joint health to maintain a healthy weight. Excess weight puts additional strain on joints, especially in weight-bearing regions such as the hips, knees, and lower back. Regular exercise, paired with a healthy diet, aids in weight management and alleviates stress.

5. Improving Circulation and Reducing Inflammation: Physical exercise improves blood circulation, ensuring that joints receive vital nutrients and oxygen. This can help decrease inflammation, which is a major cause of joint discomfort.

6. Improving Mood and Reducing Stress: - Exercise causes the release of endorphins, which are natural mood lifters. Regular physical exercise also aids in the reduction of stress, which can contribute to the experience of pain.

7. Improving Balance and Coordination: - Balance training and proprioceptive exercises, for example, increase stability and coordination. This is critical for reducing falls and injuries, especially among people who have joint discomfort.

Weight-bearing workouts such as walking, running, and weightlifting boost bone health. They increase bone density, lowering the risk of illnesses such as osteoporosis.

Adapting the Exercise to Individual Needs: - It is critical to select workouts that are suited for individual talents as well as any existing joint issues. Swimming, cycling, and yoga are ideal low-impact sports for persons suffering from joint discomfort.

Consultation and Progression: Individuals with joint discomfort should visit a healthcare physician or physical therapist before beginning or significantly altering an exercise plan. They may advise on appropriate exercises and assist in the creation of a customized program that promotes joint health.

Individuals may take proactive efforts toward improving joint health and lowering pain through natural ways by recognizing the value of regular activity.

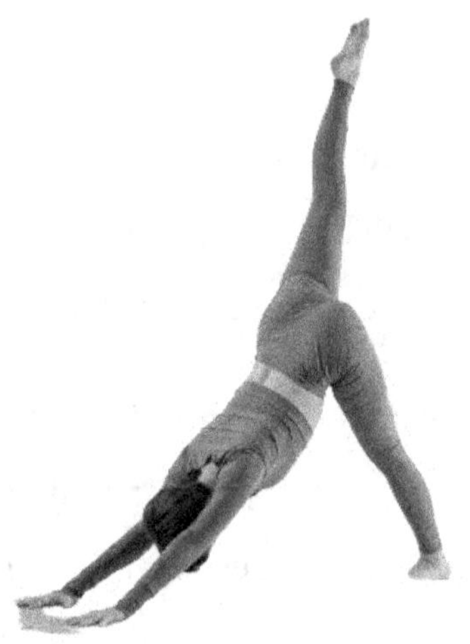

4.2 Low-Impact Exercises for Joint Pain

Individuals suffering from joint discomfort may find that including low-impact workouts into their program is quite useful. These exercises give the advantages of physical activity without putting undue strain on the joints, making them an ideal natural treatment for joint pain.

1. Swimming and Water Aerobics:

Description: Water gives buoyancy, which reduces joint impact. Swimming and water aerobics provide a full-body exercise while putting less strain on the joints. They aid in the enhancement of cardiovascular health, muscular strength, and flexibility.

Advantages: Increased range of motion, muscular tone, and cardiovascular fitness without putting load on the joints.

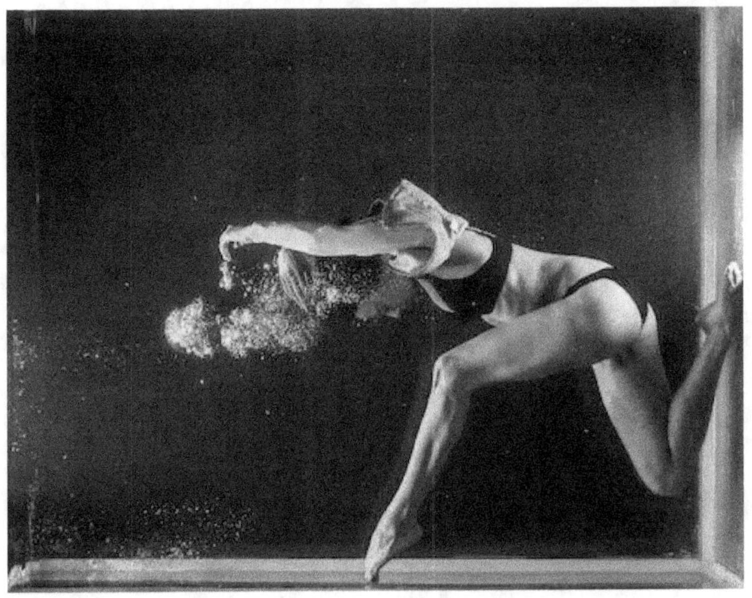

2. Cycling

Description: Cycling, whether stationary or outdoor, provides a low-impact cardiovascular workout. It works the leg muscles without placing too much strain on the knees or hips. Bike fitting is critical for comfort and joint safety.

Benefits: Improved cardiovascular health, stronger legs, and less joint strain.

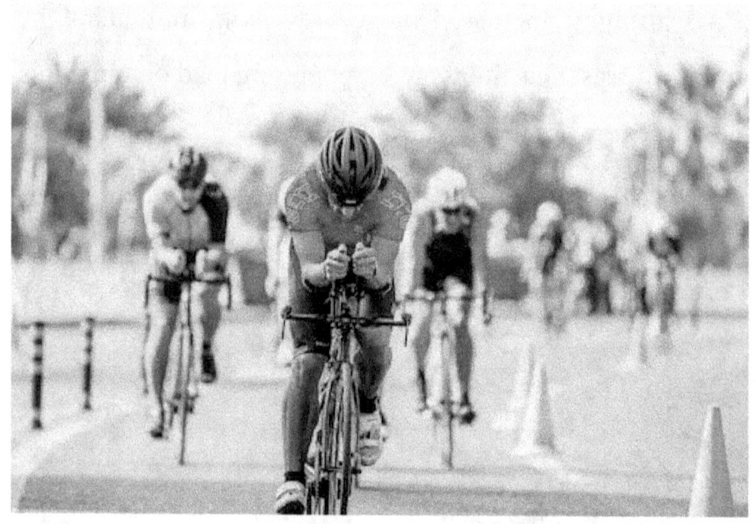

3. Elliptical Training

Description: Elliptical machines replicate the action of walking or running without the harsh effect of each stride. They target both the upper and lower body muscles, giving you a full-body exercise.

Benefits: Cardiovascular conditioning, enhanced muscle strength, and flexibility without putting strain on the joints.

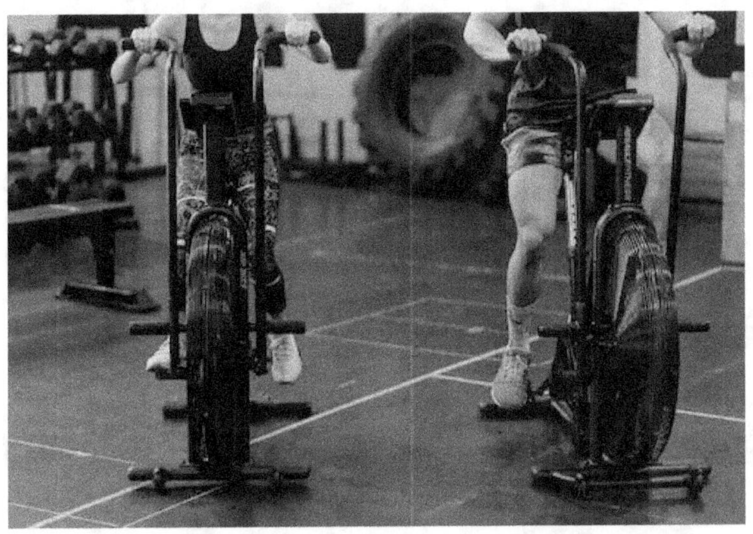

4. Yoga

Description: Yoga is a type of exercise that focuses on gentle stretching, strengthening, and balance. It encourages flexibility and relaxation, making it a good alternative for anyone suffering from joint discomfort.

Benefits include increased flexibility, better posture, greater balance, and less muscular stress.

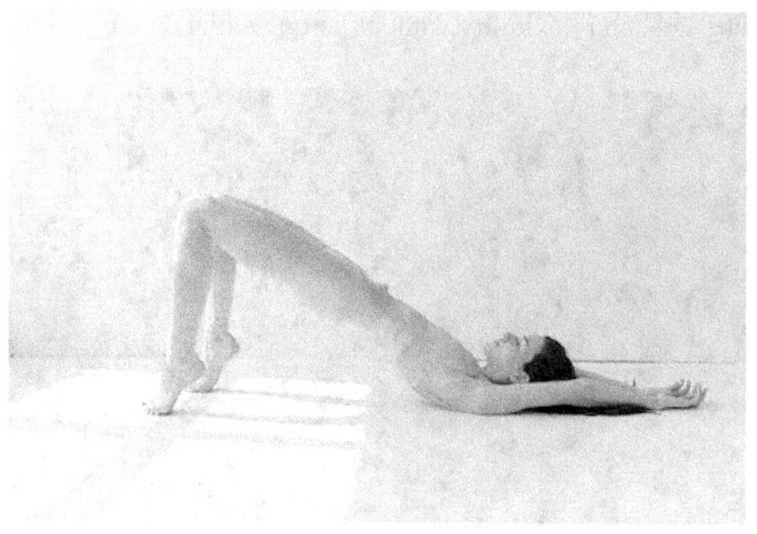

4.Tai Chi

Description: This is a leisurely, flowing practice that stresses controlled motions and deep breathing. It aids in the improvement of balance, coordination, and muscular strength, all of which are important for joint health.

Benefits: Improved balance, lower chance of falling, increased joint mobility, and less muscular tension.

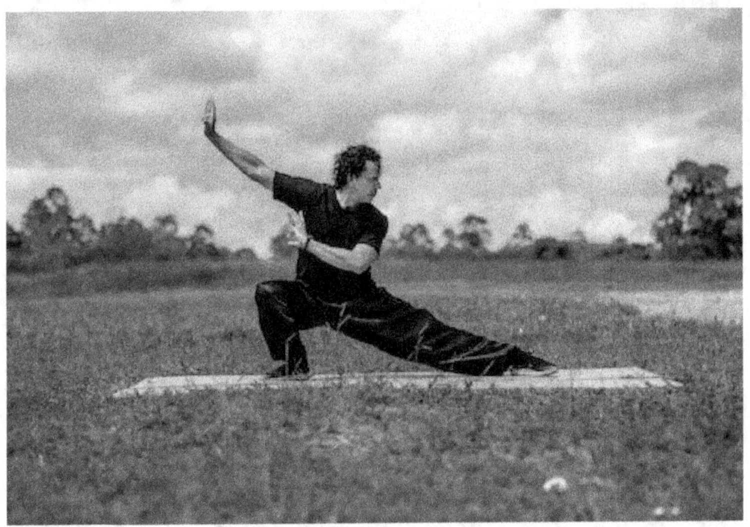

6. Pilates

Description: Pilates is a type of exercise that focuses on core strength, flexibility, and general body awareness. It provides a low-impact yet effective workout with regulated motions that target several muscle groups.

Benefits: Increased core strength, posture, flexibility, and reduced joint strain.

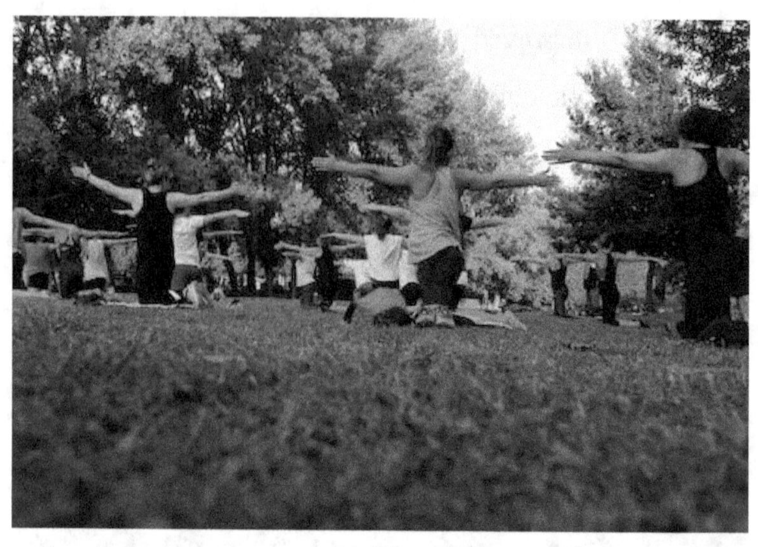

7. Resistance Band Exercises

Description: Resistance bands provide modest yet efficient resistance during exercises. They may be used for a variety of strength-training motions that target particular muscle areas without putting too much strain on the joints.

Benefits: Enhanced muscular strength, joint stability, and general joint function.

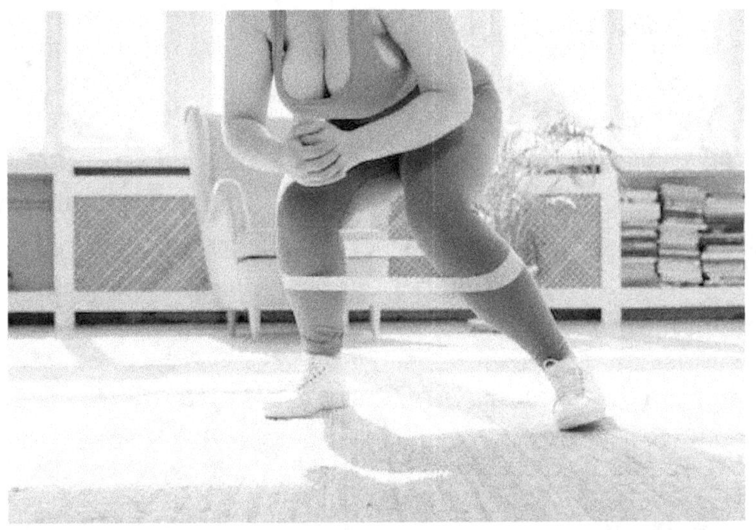

Progress and Safety: - It's critical to ease into any new fitness routine and to listen to your body. Exercises that produce pain or discomfort should be adjusted or avoided. It is strongly advised to get the advice of a healthcare physician or physical therapist regarding appropriate workouts.

Individuals can get the advantages of physical activity while avoiding stress on their joints by including low-impact exercises into their regimen, resulting in improved joint health and less discomfort.

4.3 Stretching and Strengthening Routines

Individuals seeking natural treatment from joint pain must incorporate targeted stretching and strengthening routines into their daily workout plan. These exercises aid in the improvement of flexibility, muscular support, and general joint function.

Joint Pain Stretching and Strengthening Routines

Stretching Exercises

1. Neck Stretches

Description: Tilting the head in various directions to stretch the neck muscles. This can help release stress and enhance neck mobility, which is important for people who suffer from neck and upper back discomfort.

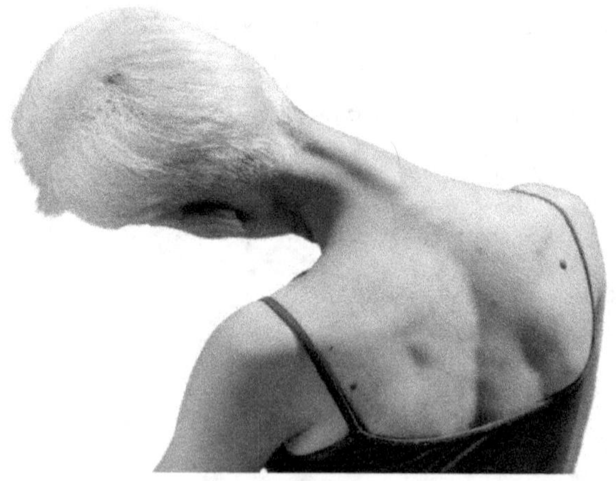

2. Shoulder Rolls and Stretches

Description: Performing stretches such as the across-the-body shoulder stretch and rotating the shoulders in circles. These exercises increase flexibility and reduce stress in the shoulders, which is useful for those who have shoulder joint pain.

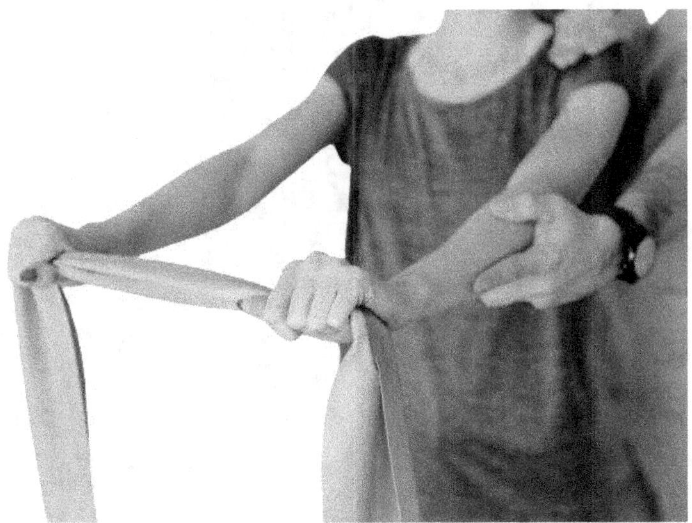

3.Chest Opener Stretch

Description: Standing with arms stretched behind you and shoulder blades squeezed together. This stretch helps to alleviate the hunched posture that can aggravate upper back and shoulder discomfort.

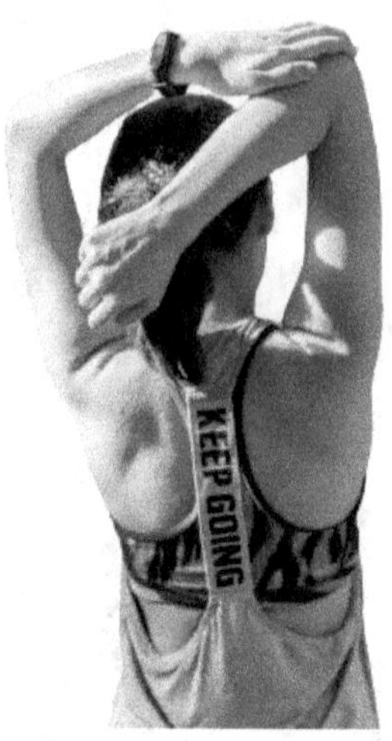

4.Back Stretches

Description: Gentle backbends, twists, and forward bends to increase spinal flexibility and relieve lower back stiffness. These stretches also work on the muscles that support the spine.

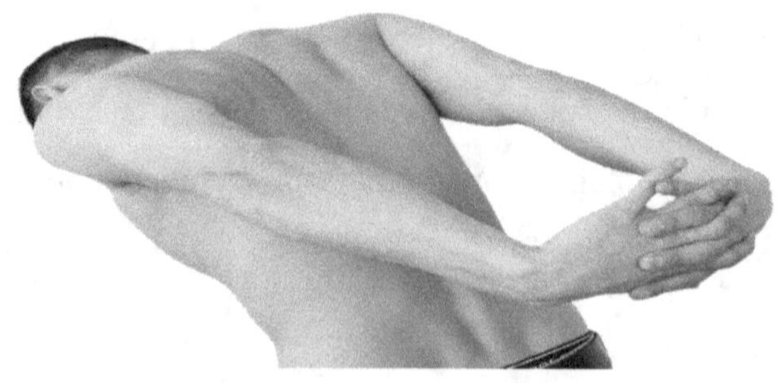

5, Hip Flexor Stretch

Description: Lunging forward to extend the front of the hip. This stretch is critical for people who have hip joint discomfort or stiffness.

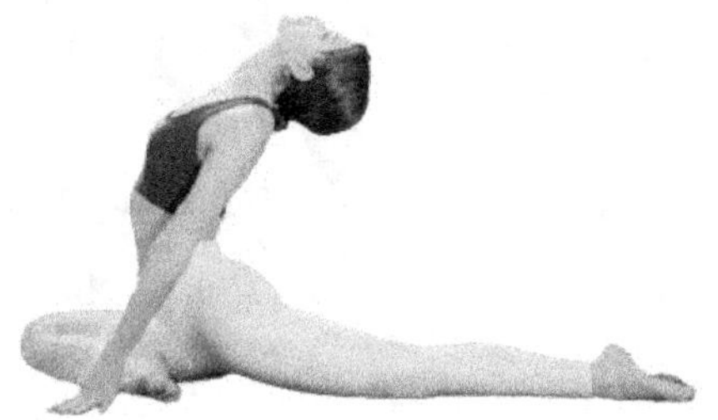

6. Quadriceps Stretch

Description: Stretching the front thigh muscles by bending one knee and holding the foot behind. This improves flexibility and relieves knee pain.

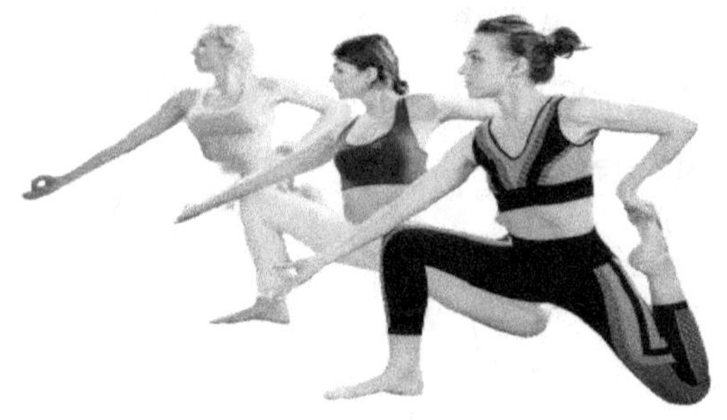

Routines for Strengthening

1. Leg Raises

Description: Lying on your back, lift one leg at a time, using your thigh muscles. This workout strengthens the quadriceps, which helps to support the knee joints.

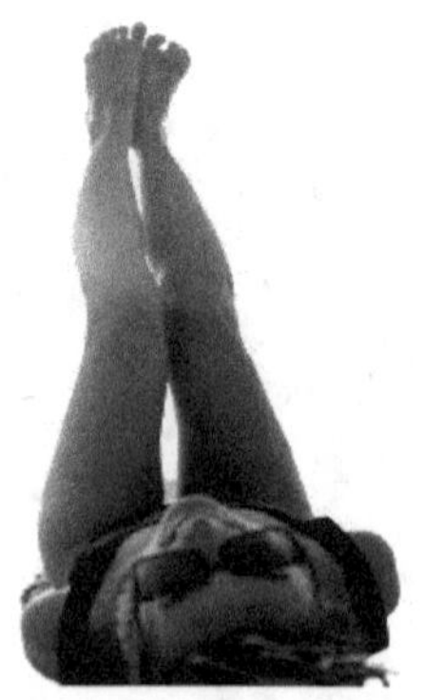

2. Bridge Exercises

Description: Lying on your back with your legs bent and your hips lifted off the ground. This strengthens the glutes and lower back, providing spine and hip stability.

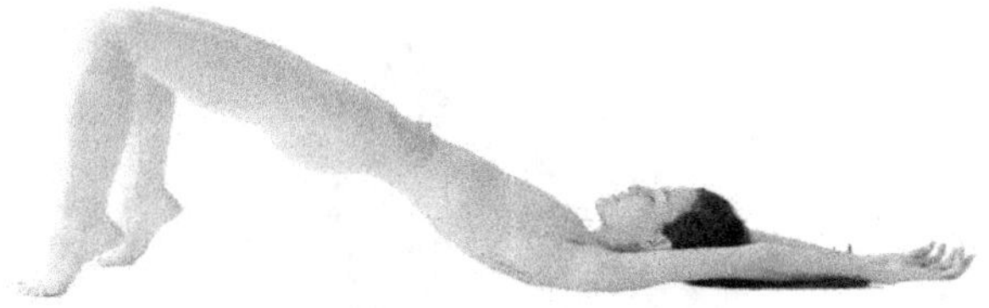

3. Planks:

Description: Standing upright on your elbows and toes. Planks activate the core muscles, giving overall stability and decreasing back pain.

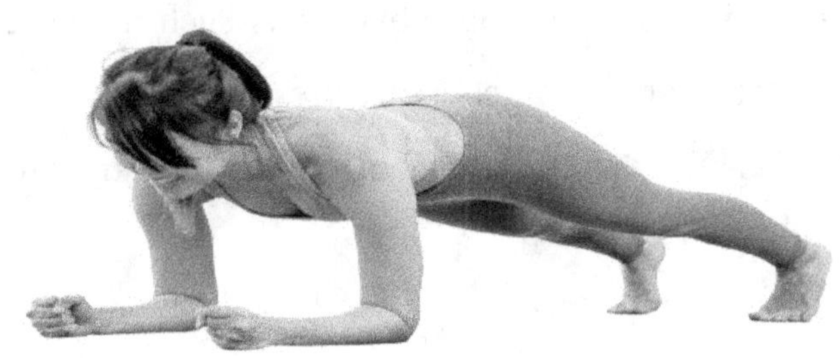

4. Exercises using Resistance Bands

Description: Resistance bands are used for workouts such as leg presses, bicep curls, and shoulder lifts. These exercises work on a variety of muscle groups to provide general strength and support.

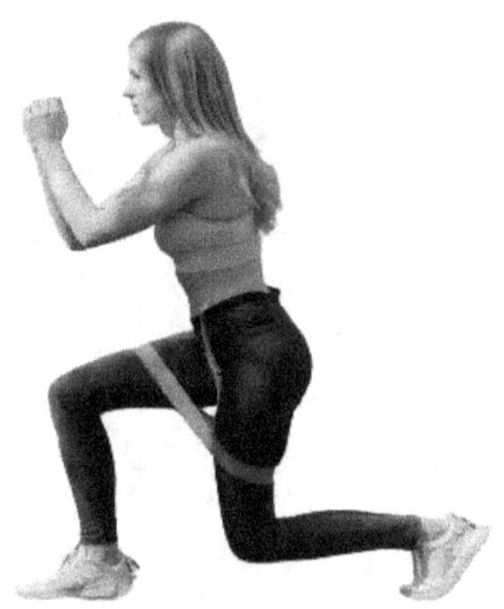

5. Gentle Weight Lifting

Description: Performing movements such as bicep curls, tricep extensions, and shoulder presses with light weights. This aids in the development of muscle strength while avoiding overexertion.

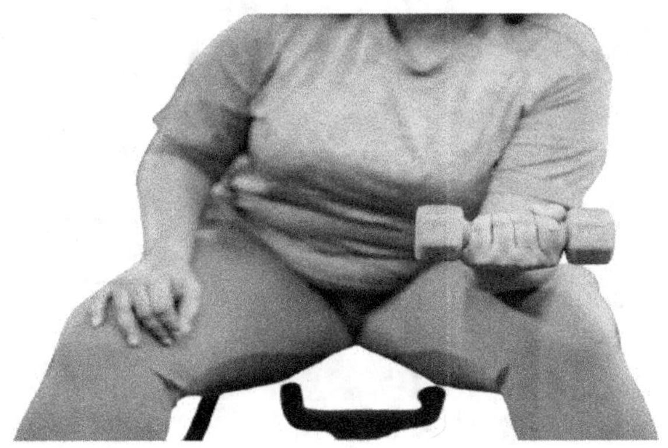

Progression and Security: - It is critical to begin with moderate stretches and exercises and gradually increase the intensity. It is critical to listen to your body and avoid any workouts that cause pain or discomfort. It is strongly advised to get the advice of a healthcare physician or physical therapist regarding proper routines.

Individuals can increase flexibility, muscular support, and general joint function by including stretching and strengthening exercises into their workout program, resulting in improved joint health and less discomfort.

Chapter 5: Lifestyle Modifications

5.1 Addressing Contributing Lifestyle Factors

Making intentional lifestyle adjustments can help greatly with joint pain management and relief. Taking care of particular issues in one's everyday life might supplement natural therapies and improve overall joint health.

1. Posture Correction

Description: Proper posture is critical for reducing stress on the spine and joints. This involves sitting with your back straight, shoulders relaxed, and your feet flat on the ground. Workplace ergonomics can also help encourage healthy posture.

2. Weight Control

Description: Maintaining a healthy weight is critical for joint health, especially in weight-bearing joints such as the knees and hips.

Excess weight puts additional strain on these joints, causing discomfort and perhaps worsening pre-existing problems such as arthritis.

3. Regular Movement pauses:

Description: Taking small pauses throughout the day to exercise and stretch will help reduce stiffness and joint discomfort. Walking, moderate stretches, or standing can enhance joint mobility and alleviate the pain associated with extended sitting.

4.Appropriate Footwear:

Description: Wearing supportive, well-fitting footwear is essential for joint health, especially for people who suffer from foot or ankle discomfort. Shoes with arch support and cushioning can assist distribute weight evenly and relieve joint pain.

5. Ergonomic modifications

Description: Making ergonomic modifications in the home and business helps reduce joint strain.

This may involve utilizing ergonomic seats, positioning the keyboard and mouse, and making sure commonly used things are conveniently accessible.

6. Balanced Workout Routine

Description: The combination of several forms of exercise, such as cardiovascular, strength training, and flexibility exercises, guarantees that all elements of joint health are addressed. Excessive pressure on individual joints can be avoided by avoiding overuse and integrating diversity.

7. Stress Reduction Techniques

Description: Stress-reduction techniques such as deep breathing exercises, meditation, or mindfulness can indirectly help joint health. High stress levels can cause physical tightness and soreness, therefore finding good relaxation strategies is critical.

8.Enough Sleep and Rest:

Description: Getting enough and good quality sleep is essential for tissue regeneration and general health.

Adequate rest promotes joint health and can help minimize pain and inflammation.

9. How to Avoid Prolonged Inactivity

Description: While rest is necessary, prolonged inactivity can cause stiffness and decreased joint mobility. Regular low-impact activities are essential for preserving joint health.

10. Hydration and Nutrition

Description: Staying hydrated and eating a well-balanced, nutrient-dense diet are critical for general health, including joint health. A balanced diet supplies vital vitamins and minerals for joint function, while hydration promotes joint lubrication.

Consultation and Progression: Individuals should consult with a healthcare practitioner or a relevant specialist before making substantial lifestyle changes. They may offer tailored guidance and ensure that planned improvements are both safe and effective.

Individuals may take proactive efforts toward controlling and reducing joint pain by addressing contributory lifestyle factors, thereby fostering improved overall joint health.

5.2 Practical Tips for Positive Changes

Practical lifestyle modifications can help substantially with joint pain management and relief. Giving tangible ideas for making good changes in everyday activities can supplement natural therapies and improve overall joint health.

Practical Suggestions for Making Positive Changes

1. Include Daily Movement

Description: Encourage low-impact exercises such as walking, swimming, and mild stretching on a regular basis. To enhance joint mobility and minimize stiffness, aim for at least 30 minutes of moderate activity most days of the week.

2. Gradual Strength Training

Description: Begin by performing light resistance workouts using bands or weights. Concentrate on main muscle groups to offer joint support and stability. Under expert supervision, gradually increase the intensity.

3. Mindful Posture Awareness

Description: Remind people to be aware of their posture throughout the day. Encourage them to sit up straight, with their shoulders aligned with their hips, and their spine in a neutral position.

4. Regular Stretching Intervals

Description: Suggest taking short breaks from work or sedentary hobbies to stretch gently. To avoid stiffness, concentrate on regions prone to stress, such as the neck, shoulders, and lower back.

5. Investigate Low-Impact Activities

Description: Swimming, cycling, and yoga are examples of joint-friendly fitness activities. These activities give cardiovascular advantages while minimizing joint stress.

6. Weight Loss Strategies

Description: Give advice on good eating habits and quantity management. Encourage them to eat nutrient-dense, whole meals and restrict processed or high-calorie snacks to help them lose weight.

7. Healthy Diet and Hydration

Description: Emphasize the value of a well-balanced diet high in anti-inflammatory foods such as fatty salmon, leafy greens, and colorful fruits and vegetables. Proper hydration promotes joint lubrication and general health.

8. Ergonomic Workspaces

Description: Provide recommendations for ergonomic workstation setup, such as correct chair height, screen arrangement, and keyboard placement. These modifications can assist to relieve tension on the neck, back, and wrists.

9. Incorporate Stress-Reduction Techniques

Description: Mindfulness practices such as deep breathing exercises, meditation, or moderate yoga are recommended. These routines can assist reduce muscular tension and increase relaxation, which can aid joint health indirectly.

10. Prioritize Quality Sleep

Description: Stress the need of developing a regular sleep pattern and generating a sleep-friendly atmosphere. Good sleep promotes tissue healing and improves overall joint health.

11. Keep a Joint-Friendly Routine

Description: Encourage people to listen to their bodies and adjust behaviors that give them pain. To avoid overuse, use a range of activities and alternate between various muscle groups.

12. Track Progress and Changes

Description: Maintain a diary to track changes in joint discomfort, mobility, and overall well-being. This can assist determine which approaches are most effective and influence future changes.

Consultation and Individualization: Emphasize the significance of consulting with a healthcare physician or appropriate specialist before making major lifestyle changes.

This guarantees that the recommended adjustments are safe and customized to the unique needs of the individual.

Individuals may take proactive efforts toward controlling and reducing joint pain by receiving practical recommendations for beneficial lifestyle adjustments, eventually fostering improved overall joint health.

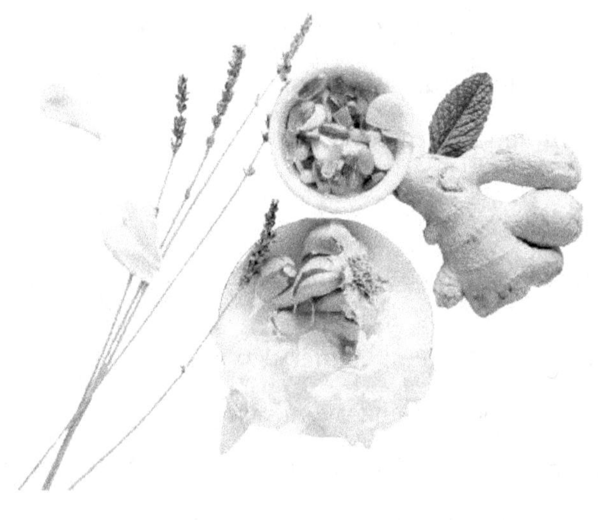

Chapter 6: Mind-Body Practices for Pain Management

6.1. Introduction to Practices (Yoga, Meditation, Breathing Techniques)

Introducing mind-body activities can be an effective way to manage and alleviate joint discomfort. This chapter examines yoga, meditation, and specific breathing methods, emphasizing their potential advantages for general joint health.

Introduction to Yoga, Meditation, and Breathing Techniques

1. Yoga

Description: Yoga is a comprehensive practice that incorporates physical postures, breathing methods, and awareness. It helps to increase flexibility, strength, and relaxation.

Benefits for Joint Health: Yoga positions gently stretch and lengthen muscles, enhancing joint mobility and decreasing stiffness.

Increased Strength: Weight-bearing yoga poses increase muscular strength while also offering joint support.

Stress Reduction: Yoga's mix of movement and awareness helps lower muscular tension and stress, which benefits joint health indirectly.

Improved Posture: Yoga promotes awareness of body alignment, which promotes improved posture and decreases joint strain.

2. Meditation:

Description: To obtain mental clarity and relaxation, meditation requires concentrated attention and regulated breathing. It can be done in a variety of ways, such as mindfulness meditation, guided visualization, or mantra-based meditation.

Pain Perception: Meditation can modify pain perception by encouraging relaxation and lowering stress levels, which helps ease joint discomfort indirectly.

Stress Reduction: Meditation helps reduce muscular tension and stress, which frequently aggravate joint pain, by soothing the mind and fostering a sense of well-being.

Better Sleep Quality: Regular meditation practice is linked to better sleep, which is essential for general joint health and pain management.

3. Pranayama (Breathing Techniques)

Description: Pranayama is a method that uses regulated breathing to increase energy and equilibrium in the body. Deep diaphragmatic breathing, alternate nostril breathing, and timed breathing exercises are examples of such strategies.

Stress Reduction: Deep, regulated breathing methods promote the body's relaxation response, lowering muscular tension and stress levels that contribute to joint discomfort.

Better Oxygenation: Proper breathing patterns guarantee an adequate flow of oxygen to muscles and joints, supporting their function and general health.

Pain Management: Mindful breathing can help people manage pain by shifting their attention and fostering a sense of calm, which provides respite from discomfort.

How to Begin Mind-Body Practices

Instruction and Instruction: Encourage individuals, especially those who are new to these activities, to seek instruction from trained teachers or use reliable resources.

Consistency is Essential: Consistent practice is required to get the full advantages of mind-body practices. Encourage them to develop a regular habit.

Adaptation and Individualization: Remind participants that practices may be tailored to their degree of comfort and physical capabilities. What is most important is their own experience and comfort.

Individuals may take proactive measures toward controlling and reducing joint pain by introducing mind-body activities such as yoga, meditation, and specific breathing methods, ultimately fostering improved overall joint health.

6.2 How They Help in Pain Management and Stress Reduction

Individuals seeking natural solutions for joint pain must first understand the importance of mind-body activities in pain management. This chapter goes into disciplines such as yoga, meditation, and specific breathing methods, looking at how they can help with pain treatment and stress reduction.

How They Aid in Pain Relief and Stress Reduction

1.Yoga

Pain Management: Through gentle stretching and regulated movements, yoga enhances joint mobility and flexibility. This helps to alleviate the stiffness and discomfort associated with joint pain.

- Weight-bearing yoga poses serve to improve muscular strength while also supporting the joints and minimizing their stress.

- Yoga's attentive nature encourages people to be present in their bodies, allowing them to listen to their limits and avoid pushing themselves beyond their comfort level, which can aggravate discomfort.

Stress Reduction: Yoga's blend of physical postures, conscious breathing, and relaxation methods activates the body's relaxation response, lowering stress chemicals such as cortisol.

- Yoga practice has been linked to decreased perceived stress and enhanced emotions of peace and well-being.

Meditation

Pain Management: Meditation modifies pain perception by diverting the focus away from discomfort. It enables people to witness pain without getting overwhelmed by it, resulting in less suffering.

- Regular meditation practice has been demonstrated to reduce pain severity and increase pain tolerance.

Stress Reduction: Mindfulness meditation teaches people to be present in the moment, letting go of anxious or unpleasant ideas. This produces a sensation of peace and tranquillity.

- Meditation affects the body's parasympathetic nervous system, which reduces stress and promotes relaxation.

3. Pranayama (Breathing Techniques)

Pain Management: - Controlled breathing techniques shift the emphasis away from pain feelings and onto the rhythm of the breath, giving the user a sense of control over their physical experience.

- Deep, diaphragmatic breathing triggers the relaxation response in the body, resulting in less muscular tension and perceived discomfort.

Stress Reduction: Using pranayama methods slows the breath, signaling the body to relax. This counteracts the body's stress reaction, resulting in a decrease in stress levels.

- Paced breathing exercises, such as alternate nostril breathing, help to build a sense of balance and equilibrium, which contributes to a more relaxed state of mind.

Using Mind-Body Techniques

Regular Practice: For maximum effect, encourage folks to include these activities into their everyday routines. Consistency is essential for obtaining the full spectrum of pain relief and stress reduction benefits.

Professional Guidance: Seek advice from trained teachers or healthcare practitioners, especially if these techniques are new to you. Proper training promotes safe and efficient implementation.

Personalization: Remind persons that these routines may be tailored to their degree of comfort and physical ability. It is critical that they respect their own bodies and experiences.

Individuals may actively manage and alleviate joint pain while simultaneously lowering stress levels by embracing mind-body activities such as yoga, meditation, and specific breathing methods, eventually encouraging greater overall joint health.

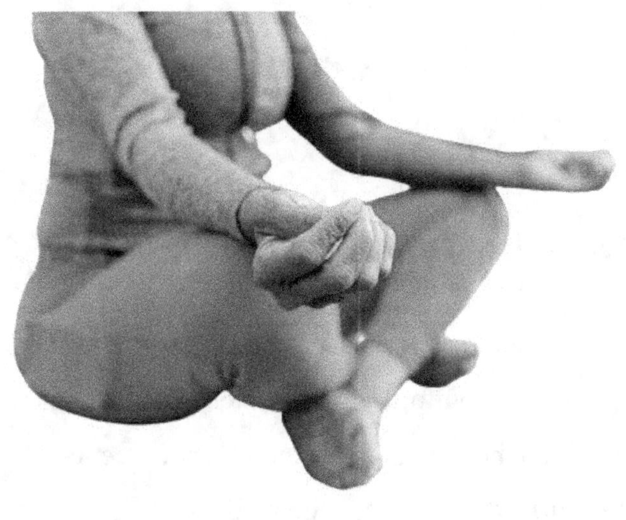

Chapter 7: Alternative Therapies

7.1 Exploration of Therapies (Acupuncture, Massage, Chiropractic Care)

Investigating alternative remedies can help you manage and relieve joint discomfort. This chapter goes into therapies such as acupuncture, massage, and chiropractic therapy, revealing information about their potential advantages for general joint health.

How They Aid in Therapy Exploration: Acupuncture, Massage, and Chiropractic Care

1. Acupuncture

Description: Acupuncture is a technique that includes inserting small needles into particular places on the body in order to enhance energy flow and facilitate healing. It is founded on the principles of traditional Chinese medicine.

Pain Relief: Acupuncture causes the body's natural painkillers, endorphins, to be released, which can give substantial relief from joint pain.

Improved Circulation: Acupuncture needle placement can enhance blood flow to afflicted regions, promoting tissue healing and lowering inflammation.

Increased Joint Mobility: Acupuncture can increase range of motion and reduce stiffness by treating particular points related to joint health.

2. Massage

Description: Massage therapy is the manipulation of soft tissues, muscles, and joints to induce relaxation, increase circulation, and relieve muscle tension.

Benefits for Joint Health

Reduced Muscle Tension: Massage methods help relieve muscle tension and promote relaxation, which benefits joint health indirectly by lowering stress on surrounding tissues.

Improved Circulation: Increased blood flow in the joints aids in nutrition delivery and waste disposal, adding to overall joint health.

Increased Flexibility: By relieving stiffness and creating more mobility, regular massage can enhance joint range of motion.

3. Chiropractic Treatment

Description: Chiropractic care is concerned with the diagnosis and treatment of musculoskeletal problems, particularly those involving the spine. Manual adjustments and spinal manipulations are frequently used.

Benefits for Joint Health

Alignment and Posture: Chiropractic treatments try to restore appropriate alignment, which can ease joint pain and improve overall posture.

Reduced Nerve Compression: Spinal misalignments can cause nerve compression, which contributes to joint pain. Chiropractic adjustments can help to relieve this stress.

Better Joint Function: Chiropractic therapy can improve joint function by restoring appropriate spinal alignment, decreasing pain and stiffness.

Investigating Alternative Therapies

Professional Counseling: Stress the significance of receiving therapy from qualified and experienced practitioners. It guarantees that people receive safe, effective treatment that is adapted to their personal requirements.

Integration with Other Treatments: Alternative treatments can be used in conjunction with other natural cures such as dietary modifications and exercise. Encourage people to talk to their healthcare practitioners about possible synergies.

Regular Treatment Schedule: Consistent and regular sessions are frequently required to get the full advantages of alternative therapies. Encourage people to develop a treatment plan that fits their schedule and goals.

Individuals can take proactive efforts toward treating and reducing joint pain by investigating alternative therapies such as acupuncture, massage, and chiropractic therapy, eventually fostering improved overall joint health.

7.2 Potential Benefits for Joint Pain Relief

Investigating alternative therapies provides a comprehensive approach to controlling and reducing joint pain. This chapter goes into therapies such as acupuncture, massage, and chiropractic therapy, revealing important information about their potential advantages for general joint health.

Acupuncture, Massage, and Chiropractic Care Have Potential Benefits for Joint Pain Relief

1. Acupuncture

Pain Relieving: Acupuncture activates the body's inherent pain-relieving processes. It causes the production of endorphins, which are potent analgesics, by targeting certain acupuncture sites. This results in great joint pain alleviation.

Reduction of Inflammation: Acupuncture has been demonstrated to alter the body's inflammatory response. It can relieve pain and aid healing by lowering inflammation around afflicted joints.

Increased Blood Flow: Inserting acupuncture needles enhances blood flow to the targeted locations. This increased blood flow promotes tissue healing and alleviates stiffness and soreness.

2. Massage

Reduction of muscular Tension: Massage therapy tackles muscular tension and stiffness, which frequently contribute to joint discomfort. It indirectly benefits joint health by relieving stress in surrounding muscles.

Better Circulation: Massage methods improve blood flow, which helps supply nutrients and oxygen to joint tissues. This benefits their general health and may help with pain alleviation.

Endorphin Release: Massage, like acupuncture, stimulates the release of endorphins. Individuals suffering from joint discomfort will benefit from this natural process, which delivers a sensation of relaxation and pain reduction.

3. Chiropractic Treatment

Spinal Alignment: Chiropractic adjustments aim to correct spinal alignment. This can reduce joint pain by relieving strain on nerves and supporting overall musculoskeletal health.

Posture Improvement: Spinal misalignments can cause poor posture, which can contribute to joint pain. Chiropractic therapy tackles these concerns by establishing improved posture and alignment.

Improved Joint Function: Chiropractic therapy can enhance joint function by treating spinal misalignments. This reduces pain and stiffness, allowing people to move more easily.

Consultation and Evaluation: Encourage persons to seek advice from skilled practitioners in each therapy. A comprehensive assessment ensures that therapies are matched to their unique requirements and situations.

Integration with Other Remedies: Alternative treatments can be used with other natural remedies such as dietary modifications and exercise programs. To build a complete approach to joint health, encourage open communication with healthcare professionals.

Consistency and Commitment: Regular and consistent sessions are frequently required to get the full advantages of alternative therapies. Encourage them to commit to a treatment plan that is in line with their aspirations.

Individuals can actively participate in controlling and reducing joint pain by investigating alternative therapies such as acupuncture, massage, and chiropractic therapy, eventually fostering improved overall joint health.

Chapter 8: Home Remedies and DIY Treatments

8.1 Easy-to-Follow Recipes for Topical Treatments

A critical element of joint pain care is providing clients with realistic, at-home alternatives. This chapter examines simple topical therapy formulations, offering users with efficient solutions to alleviate joint discomfort using natural materials.

Topical Treatment Recipes for Beginners

1. Natural Balms

Ingredients: beeswax, coconut oil, essential oils (eucalyptus, lavender), arnica oil.

Preparation: Melt together beeswax and coconut oil. A few drops of essential oils and arnica oil should be added. To solidify, pour the mixture into molds.

Application: Massage the balm into the afflicted joints. Massage lightly to relieve pain. Beeswax and essential oils work together to create a relaxing and warming sensation.

2. Epsom Salt Compression

Ingredients: Epsom salt, warm water, and a clean towel.

Preparation: In warm water, dissolve Epsom salt. Soak the cloth in the solution and wring it out.

Usage: Apply the warm compress to the afflicted joint. Allow it to sit for 15-20 minutes. Epsom salt relaxes muscles and relieves joint pain.

3. Turmeric Paste

Ingredients: Turmeric powder and water.

Preparation: Make a paste using turmeric powder and water.

Use: Apply the paste to the afflicted region. Leave it on for 15-20 minutes before rinsing. Turmeric's anti-inflammatory benefits are well recognized.

4. Salve with ginger and cayenne pepper

Ingredients: fresh ginger, cayenne pepper, olive oil, and beeswax.

Preparation: Over low heat, infuse olive oil with grated ginger and cayenne pepper. Strain the oil and combine it with the melted beeswax.

Usage: Apply the salve to the afflicted joint. Warming comfort is provided by the combination of ginger and cayenne pepper.

5. Soak in Apple Cider Vinegar

Ingredients: apple cider vinegar and warm water.

Preparation: In a basin, combine equal parts apple cider vinegar and warm water.

Application: Soak for 15-20 minutes the afflicted joint. Apple cider vinegar may aid in the reduction of inflammation and the relief of joint discomfort.

Considerations for Do-It-Yourself Treatments

Patch Test: Encourage people to undertake a patch test before using any new topical medicine to make sure they don't have an allergic response.

Consistency: Remind people to utilize these therapies on a frequent basis for the greatest outcomes. Consistent application is essential for reaping the maximum effects.

Consultation: Before attempting new treatments, consumers should check with their healthcare professional, especially if they have allergies or underlying medical concerns.

Individuals may actively engage in their own joint pain management by giving easy-to-follow recipes for topical therapies that use natural components that provide calming relief.

8.2 Techniques like Hot/Cold Therapy, Epsom Salt Baths

It is critical to provide folks with accessible and effective at-home remedies while dealing with joint discomfort.

This chapter delves into treatments such as hot/cold therapy and Epsom salt baths, offering individuals practical ways to relieve discomfort and enhance joint health.

Methods such as Hot/Cold Therapy and Epsom Salt Baths

1. Hot and Cold Therapy

Description: Hot and cold treatment includes applying heat and cold to the afflicted joint alternately.

Use Case:

Hot Compress: For 15-20 minutes, use a hot water bottle, heating pad, or warm cloth to the joint. This improves blood circulation, relaxes muscles, and reduces stiffness.

Cold Compress: For 10-15 minutes, apply a cold pack or a bag of frozen vegetables wrapped in a towel to the joint. Cold treatment relieves pain by reducing inflammation and numbing the affected region.

Timing: Alternate between hot and cold therapy for 30-40 minutes, beginning and finishing with heat. This can be done twice a day.

Caution: Always use a barrier, such as a towel, to protect your skin from direct contact with high heat. Avoid putting cold packs directly on your skin.

Epsom Salt Baths

Description: Epsom salt, a magnesium and sulfate compound, is well recognized for its medicinal effects.

Planning

Ingredients: 1-2 cups Epsom salt and warm water.

Application: Soak the afflicted joint in a warm bath with Epsom salt for 15-20 minutes.

Advantages

Muscle Relaxation: The magnesium in Epsom salt relaxes muscles, which can help ease joint pain indirectly.

Reduced Inflammation: The magnesium and warm water work together to lessen inflammation around the joint.

Improved Blood Circulation: Epsom salt can aid in the supply of nutrients and oxygen to the joints by improving blood flow.

Frequency: Epsom salt baths can be taken 2-3 times each week, or as needed.

Considerations for Do-It-Yourself Treatments

Water Temperature: Make sure the water temperature for hot treatment is warm but not scorching. Use a frozen cold pack or a bag of ice wrapped in a towel for cold treatment.

Consultation: Encourage people to talk to their doctor before starting any new therapy, especially if they have circulatory problems or other medical concerns.

Comfort and Relaxation: Remind patients to establish a relaxing environment during their treatments, as this can improve the entire therapeutic experience.

Individuals may actively participate in their own joint pain treatment by introducing techniques such as hot/cold therapy and Epsom salt baths into their regimen, using accessible and natural means to find comfort.

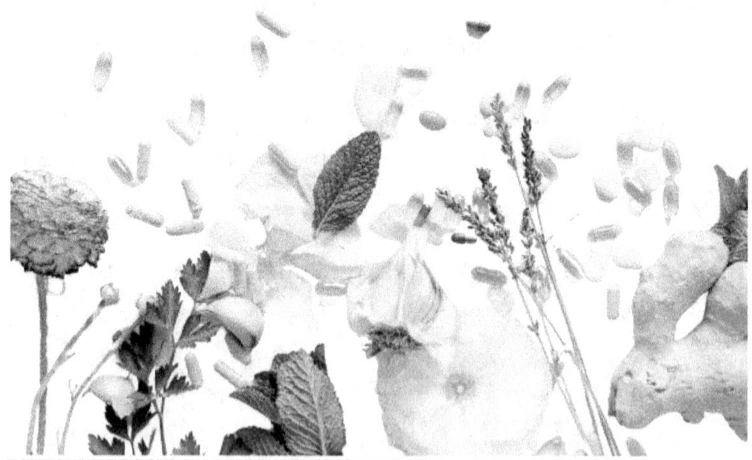

Chapter 9: Case Studies and Testimonials

9.1 Real-Life Success Stories with Natural Remedies

Real-life success stories may be great motivators and sources of inspiration for anyone seeking joint pain alleviation. This chapter contains case studies and testimonies from people who have successfully treated joint pain using natural medicines.

Real-Life Natural Remedies Success Stories

1. Case Study 1: Sarah's Turmeric and Yoga Journey

Context: Sarah, a 45-year-old lady, has been suffering from persistent knee discomfort caused by osteoarthritis. She began incorporating turmeric into her daily diet and began doing yoga on a regular basis.

Result: Sarah noticed a considerable reduction in pain and stiffness over a period of many months.

Her everyday life was revolutionized by the anti-inflammatory qualities of turmeric, paired with the flexibility and strength she developed from yoga.

Takeaway: Sarah's experience demonstrates the power of natural therapies and lifestyle modifications in treating and even relieving arthritis-related joint pain.

2. Testimonial 1: John's Fish Oil Supplement Experience

Background: John, a 50-year-old male, has been suffering from rheumatoid arthritis-related joint discomfort in his hands and wrists. He added Omega-3 fatty acid supplements, largely derived from fish oil, to his daily regimen.

Result: John noted a considerable reduction in inflammation and discomfort after a few weeks. The Omega-3 fatty acids were an excellent supplement to his joint health program.

Takeaway: John's testimony highlights the potential benefits of adopting targeted supplements, such as fish oil, into a joint health program.

3. Case Study 2: Maria's Acupuncture Success

Background: Maria, a 55-year-old lady, has been suffering from persistent lower back discomfort caused by arthritis and muscular strain. She sought out qualified acupuncturists on a regular basis.

Result: Maria's pain levels decreased noticeably over the course of many months. Acupuncture gave her a non-invasive and efficient approach to manage her joint pain.

Takeaway: Maria's case study demonstrates the potential of alternative therapies such as acupuncture in relieving joint discomfort.

Thoughts on Case Studies and Testimonials

Diverse Perspectives: Include case studies and testimonies from people of all ages, backgrounds, and forms of joint pain. This helps readers to relate to a wide range of experiences.

Expert Guidance: Stress the significance of getting expert advice before making major modifications to one's treatment plan.

Personalized Approaches: Emphasize the fact that what works for one person may not work for another. Encourage readers to try out different cures to see what works best for them.

Individuals can find hope and encouragement to research natural therapies for their own joint pain management by sharing real-life success stories.

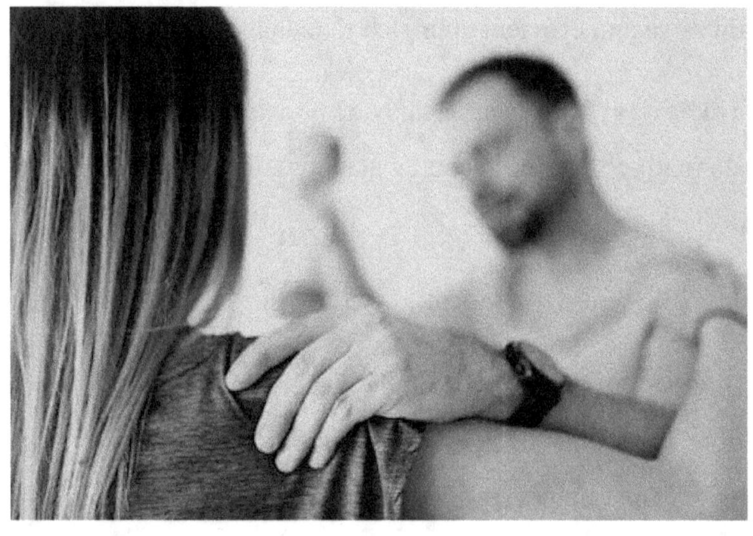

Chapter 10: Empowering Adults for Joint Pain Relief

10.1 Key Takeaways

The ultimate purpose of this book is to provide individuals with the knowledge and skills they need to take control of their joint health. This last chapter summarizes the most crucial elements for efficient joint pain management from the whole book.

Key Joint Pain Relief Takeaways

1. Recognizing Joint Pain

- Arthritis, overuse, injuries, and other conditions can all contribute to joint discomfort.

- It is critical to distinguish between acute and chronic joint pain in order to manage it effectively.

2. Joint Health Diet and Nutrition

- A healthy diet rich in anti-inflammatory foods such as fatty fish, curcumin, and berries is beneficial to joint health.

- Joint health supplements such as Omega-3 fatty acids, glucosamine, and chondroitin might be beneficial.

3. Herbal Supplements and Remedies

- Natural supplements such as ginger, Boswellia, and devil's claw can help relieve joint discomfort.

- Consideration should be given to dosage recommendations and potential interactions.

4. Physical Activity and Exercise

- Maintaining joint health requires regular, low-impact exercise as well as specific stretching and strengthening programs.

5. Lifestyle Changes:

- Addressing variables such as posture and weight control helps to improve overall joint health.

- Making healthy lifestyle adjustments can help lessen joint discomfort dramatically.

6. Mind-Body Techniques for Pain Management

- Yoga, meditation, and deep breathing methods help with pain management and stress reduction.

7. Alternative Therapies

- Acupuncture, massage, and chiropractic therapy all have the ability to relieve joint discomfort.

8. Home Remedies and Do-It-Yourself Treatments

- Simple topical treatment formulations, as well as procedures like hot/cold therapy and Epsom salt baths, make relief more accessible.

9. Real-World Success Stories

- Case studies and testimonials indicate the efficacy of natural therapies in the treatment of joint pain.

Personalized Approach: Encourage people to personalize their treatments and lifestyle modifications to their own requirements and preferences.

Consultation with Healthcare Providers: Stress the need of speaking with healthcare providers before making major modifications to treatment plans.

Patience and Consistency: Remind folks that results may take time, and that constant effort is required to get the full advantages of natural therapies.

Individuals may take proactive actions toward improving joint health by internalizing these important principles, eventually finding relief and empowerment in their road to a pain-free life.

10.2 Encouragement for Proactive Joint Health

The ultimate purpose of this book is to empower individuals to take care of their joint health. This last chapter is a call to action, offering encouragement and direction for proactive joint health.

Support for Proactive Joint Health

1. Recognizing the Journey

- Recognize that controlling joint pain is a journey, and that improvement may be slow.

- Recognize minor successes and progress along the road.

2. Customized Approach

- Enable people to personalize natural therapies and lifestyle adjustments to their own requirements and preferences.

- Emphasize the significance of determining what works best for each individual.

3. Consultation with Healthcare Professionals

- Encourage open dialogue with healthcare providers. Individuals can then make educated judgments concerning their joint health.

- Routine check-ins with healthcare specialists can give crucial insight and treatment plan changes.

4. Patience and Consistency

- Emphasize that outcomes may not be instant, and that consistency is essential. Natural therapies and good behaviors should be used on a regular basis to get long-term healing.

- Patience is essential in the process of determining the most effective joint pain management solutions.

5. Lifestyle as a Basis

- Emphasize the effect of lifestyle on joint health. Encourage people to make healthy adjustments in their posture, food, exercise, and stress management.

- Remind them that these lifestyle changes are essential for long-term joint health.

6. Mind-Body Relationship

- Stress the significance of techniques such as yoga, meditation, and deep breathing. These treatments not only alleviate pain but also promote mental health.

- A mind-body approach that is balanced adds to total joint health and quality of life.

7. Rejoice in Progress

- Encourage people to keep track of their improvement, whether it's greater mobility, pain relief, or general well-being.

- Recognizing accomplishments encourages a good attitude and motivates continued dedication to joint health.

Lifetime Commitment

- Emphasize that joint health is a lifetime commitment. Consistent attention and care for joint health contribute to long-term alleviation and well-being.

Individuals are enabled to take ownership of their well-being and begin on a journey towards a life with decreased joint pain and increased overall quality of life by giving encouragement and direction for proactive joint health.

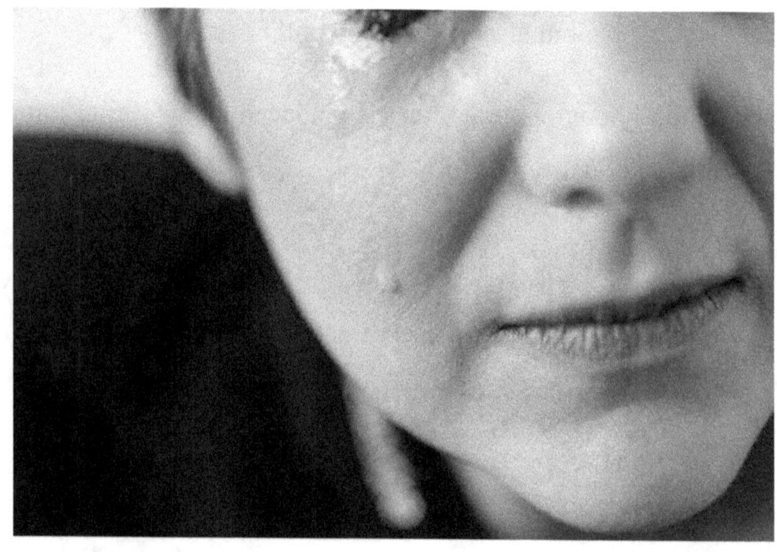

Additional Resources and References

Reputable Sources, Websites, and Recommended Reading

It is critical to provide them with trustworthy sources of knowledge and additional reading materials as they progress toward better joint health. This section contains a carefully chosen selection of reliable sources, websites, and suggested readings on joint health and natural therapies.

Reliable Resources

1. National Institutes of Health (NIH) - Arthritis, Musculoskeletal Diseases, and Skin Diseases: This government organization offers in-depth and well-researched information on many forms of arthritis and joint problems. Their website provides both patients and healthcare professionals with articles, publications, and tools.

2. The Arthritis Foundation: A renowned non-profit organization committed to assisting people suffering from arthritis. Their website has a plethora of information about various forms of arthritis, therapies, and lifestyle management.

3. Mayo Clinic: A well-known medical facility recognized for providing dependable and simple-to-understand health information. The Mayo Clinic website has a section dedicated to joint pain that covers causes, symptoms, and treatment options.

Websites

1. PubMed: A database of peer-reviewed medical research publications. Scholarly publications on joint health, natural therapies, and other relevant subjects may be found.

2. Arthritis Health Center on WebMD: WebMD offers an easy-to-use platform with articles, expert advice, and videos on arthritis and joint health. It contains a lot of information for anyone who want to understand and treat joint discomfort.

3. MedlinePlus-Joint Disorders: The National Library of Medicine's website offers a wealth of information about joint diseases, including treatment choices and preventative techniques.

Suggested Reading

1. Jason Theodosakis, Brenda Adderly, and Barry Fox's "The Arthritis Cure": This book delves at natural ways to arthritis management, such as dietary changes and supplements.

2. Yoga for Arthritis: The Complete Guide by Loren Fishman and Ellen Saltonstall's: An in-depth look at utilizing yoga as a supplemental therapy for arthritis and joint discomfort.

3. The Inflammation Syndrome: Your Nutrition Plan for Great Health, Weight Loss, and Pain-Free Living" by Jack Challem: This book explains how diet may affect inflammation, which is a major cause of joint discomfort.

Individual Preferences: Encourage folks to investigate various resources and identify those that correspond to their learning style and preferences.

Continual Learning: Stress the significance of continued education and remaining current on joint health advancements.

Consultation with Healthcare Providers: Remind folks to consult with their healthcare provider about any new treatments or methods to ensure they are appropriate for their personal health requirements.

Individuals have access to accurate information and may continue their journey towards better joint health with confidence and understanding thanks to a well-chosen list of reputable sources, websites, and suggested readings.

Conclusion

As you complete the last chapter of this inspiring adventure, you hold the keys to a future free of joint pain. This book was written with one goal in mind: to provide you with knowledge, techniques, and natural cures that will put you in control of your own health.

You now have the knowledge to differentiate between acute and chronic pain, insight into the factors that may be impacting you, and a rich tapestry of natural treatments that may improve your everyday life.

Remember that your path to joint pain treatment is not a solitary one. You are part of a community of people who want the same thing as you, and your struggles and victories will motivate others to take care of their own health.

You are nourishing your body in a way that allows it to recover when you eat a balanced diet, add anti-inflammatory foods, and investigate the advantages of supplements. Exercise strengthens not just your joints but also your will to live a pain-free life.

Lifestyle changes and mind-body activities are not just ideas; they are strong tools that will assist you in reclaiming your energy. Alternative treatments provide you with a plethora of possibilities, each of which may hold the secret to your own recovery path.

You can find accessible, natural, and astonishingly efficient cures in your own house. In this journey, hot/cold therapy and Epsom salt baths become your allies, always on hand to bring relief.

Above all, remember that the tales recounted inside these pages are just the beginning. You write your own story, and every decision you make, every stride you take toward a life free of joint pain, demonstrates your power and dedication.

So, go on with confidence, knowing that you've made an important step toward a pain-free future. Your adventure continues, and the finest chapters are still to come. Accept this newfound information, use it with purpose, and take a brave step into a life of energy, freedom, and joy.

Your future is pain-free and full of potential.

Workout Planner

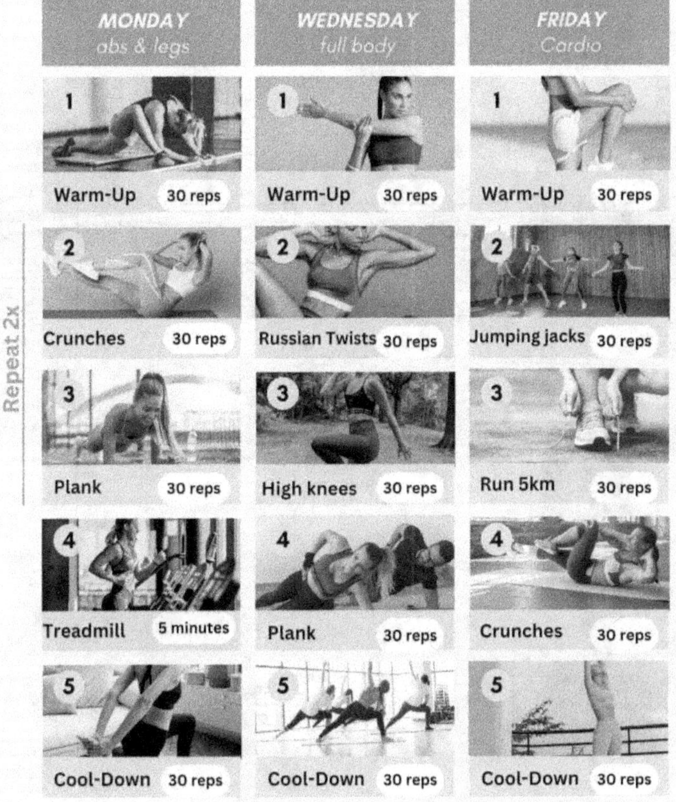

WORKOUT PLANNER

	EXERCISE	GOAL
MON DAY		
WEDNES DAY		
FRI DAY		

WORKOUT PLANNER

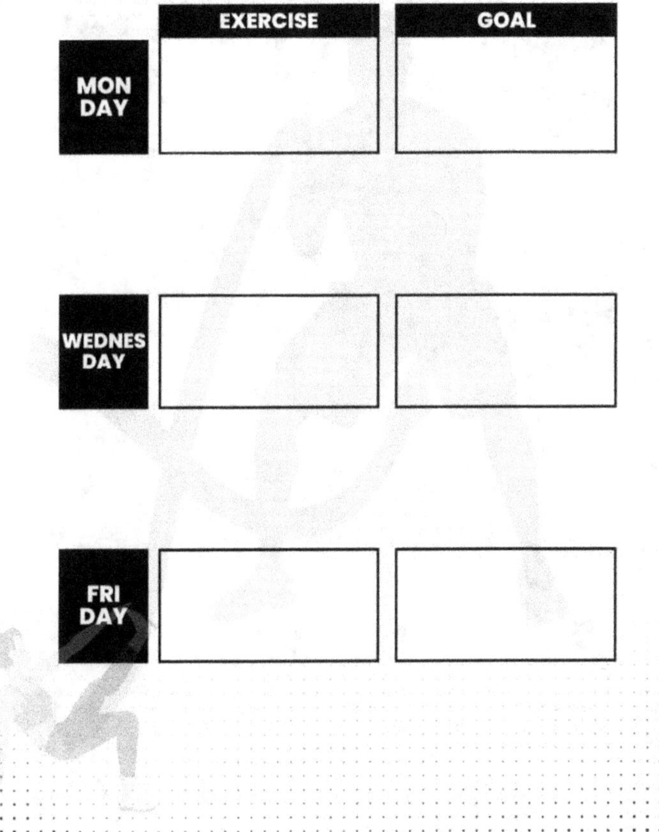

WORKOUT PLANNER

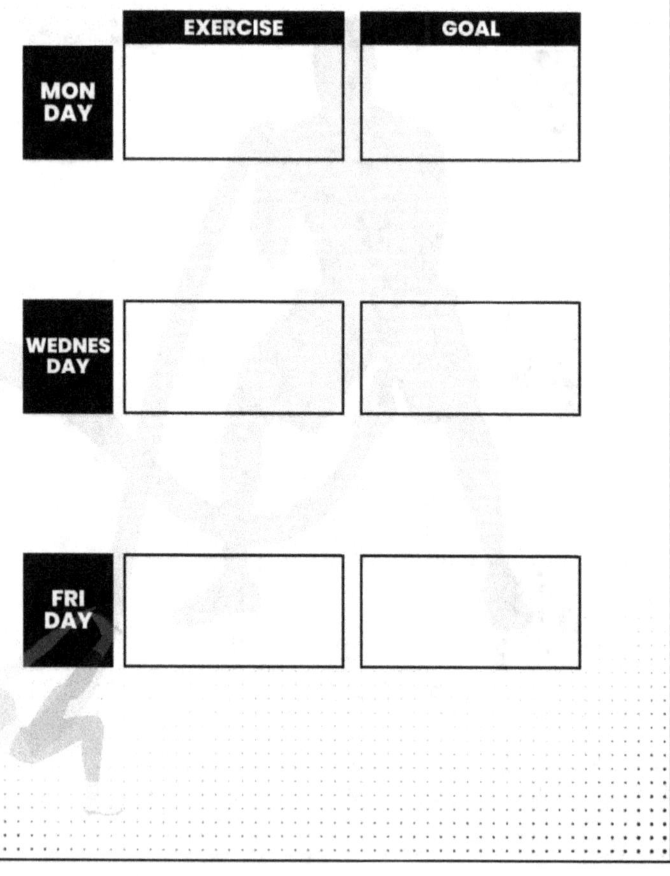

	EXERCISE	GOAL
MON DAY		
WEDNES DAY		
FRI DAY		

WORKOUT PLANNER

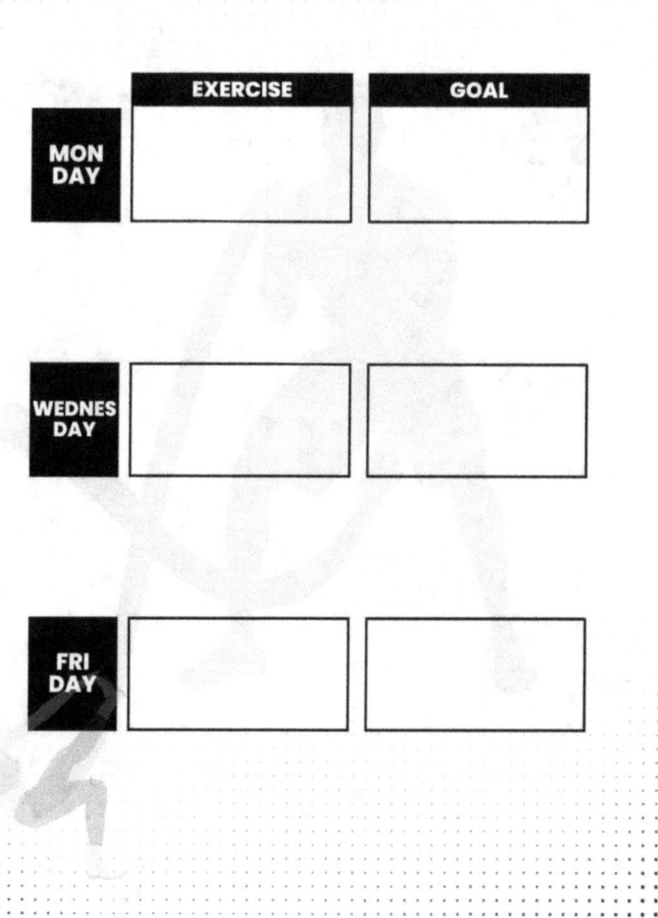

WORKOUT PLANNER

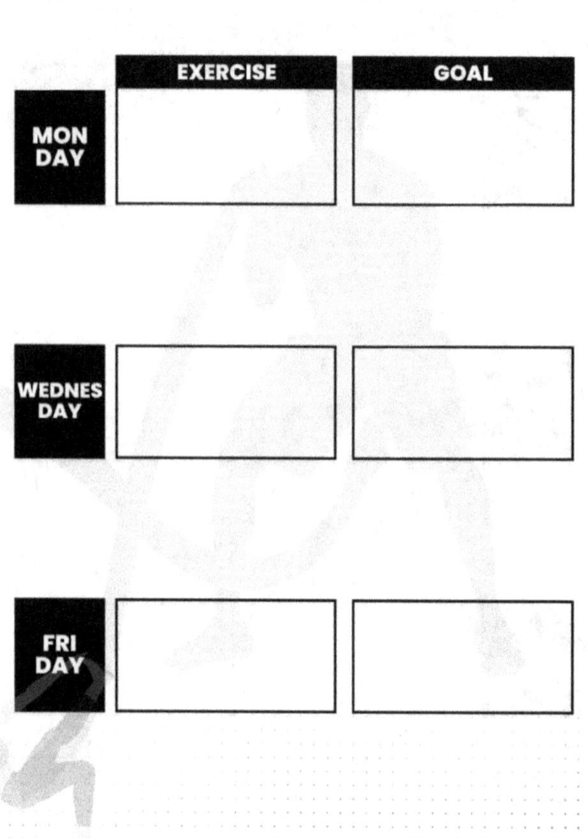

WORKOUT PLANNER

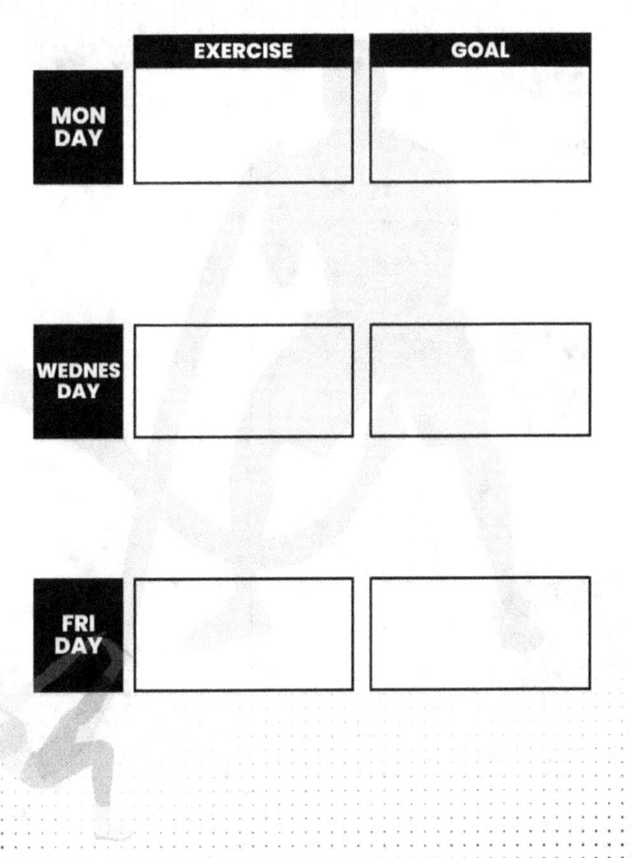

WORKOUT PLANNER

	EXERCISE	GOAL
MON DAY		
WEDNES DAY		
FRI DAY		

WORKOUT PLANNER

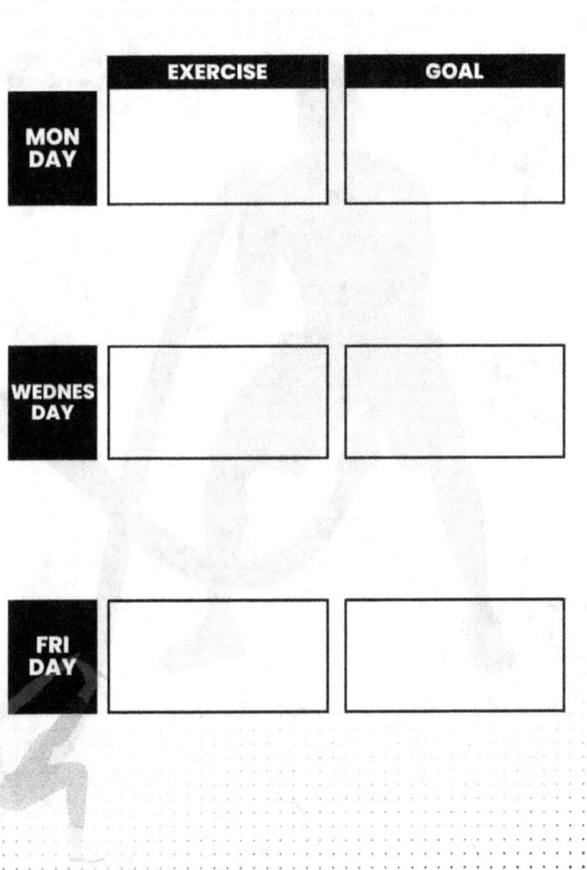

WORKOUT PLANNER

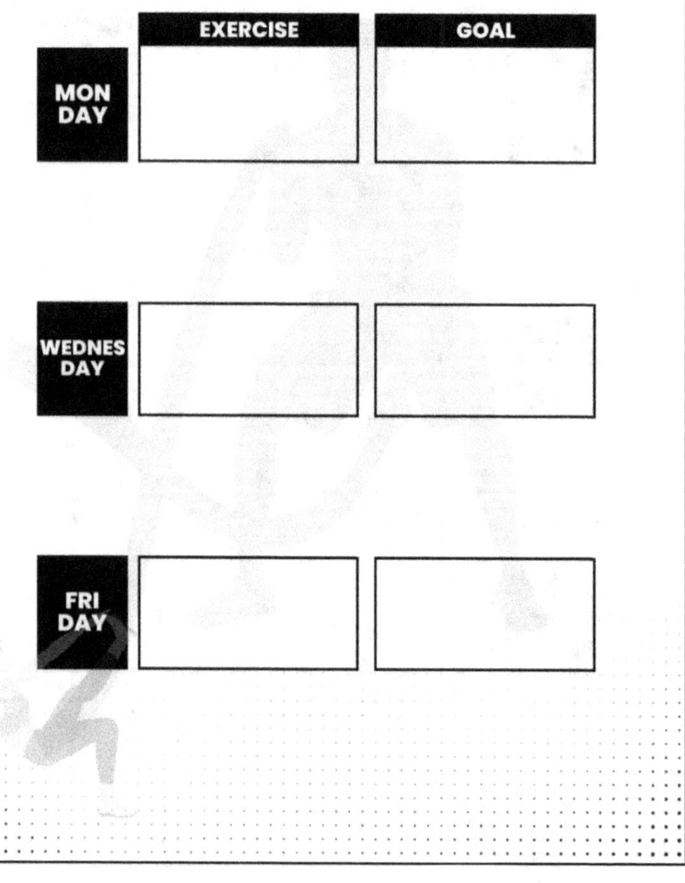

WORKOUT PLANNER

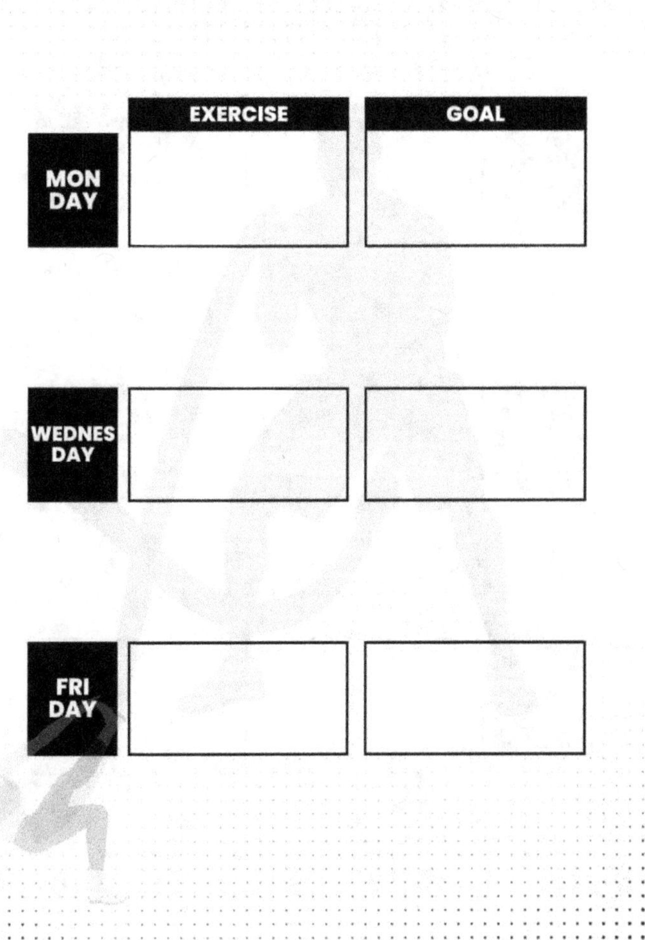

	EXERCISE	GOAL
MON DAY		
WEDNES DAY		
FRI DAY		

WORKOUT PLANNER

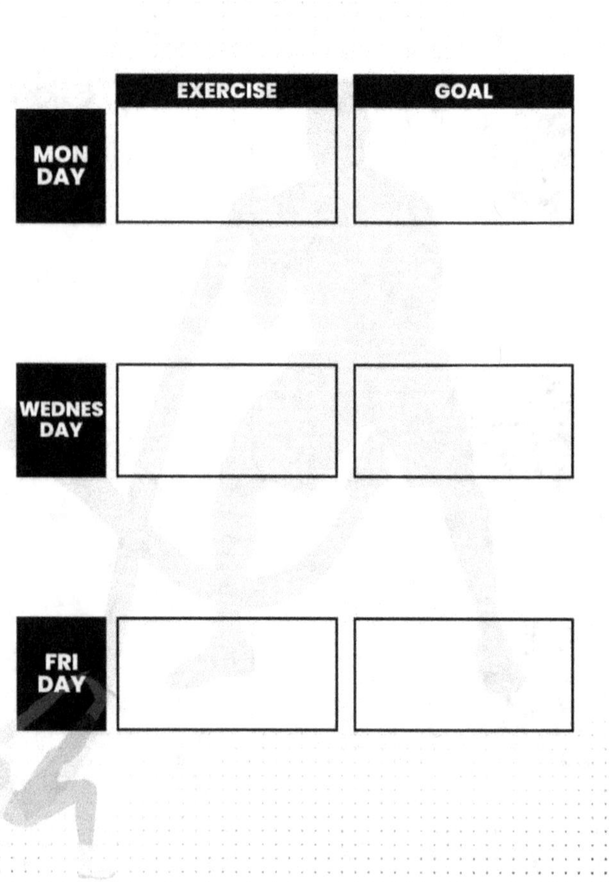

WORKOUT PLANNER

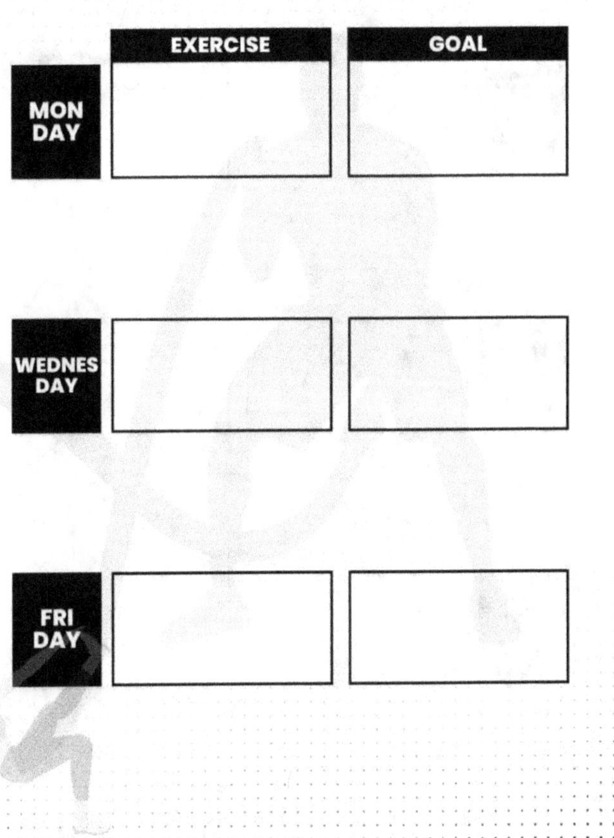

WORKOUT PLANNER

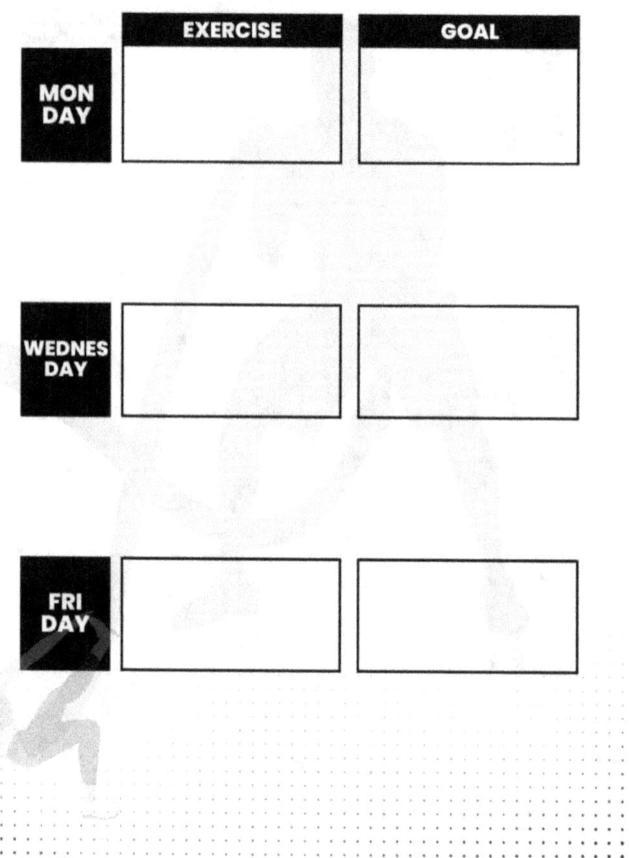

WORKOUT PLANNER

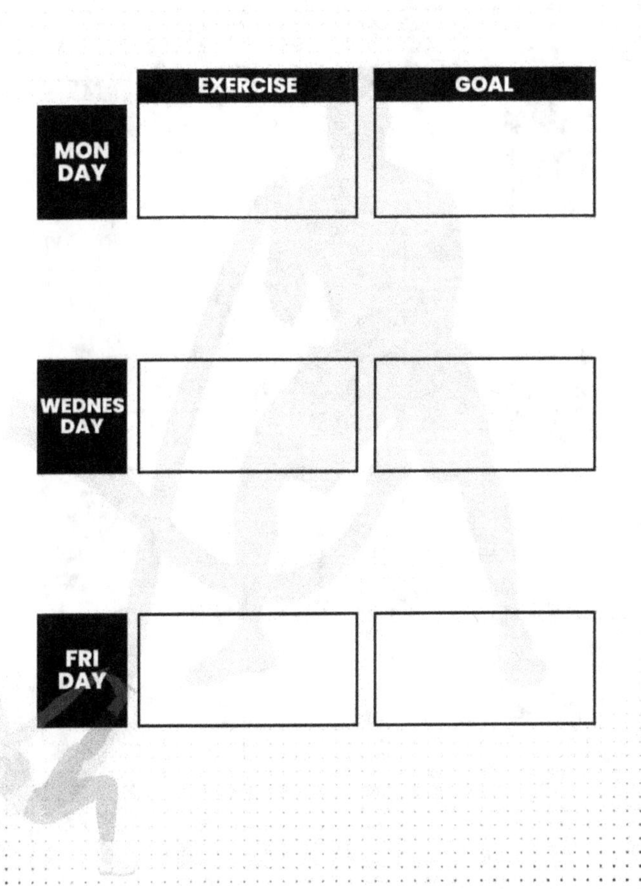

WORKOUT PLANNER

	EXERCISE	GOAL
MON DAY		
WEDNES DAY		
FRI DAY		

WORKOUT PLANNER

	EXERCISE	GOAL
MON DAY		
WEDNES DAY		
FRI DAY		

WORKOUT PLANNER

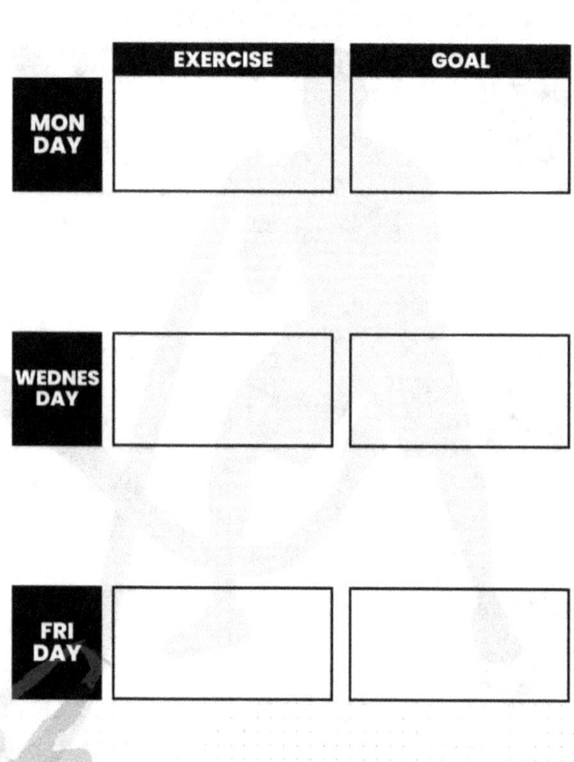

WORKOUT PLANNER

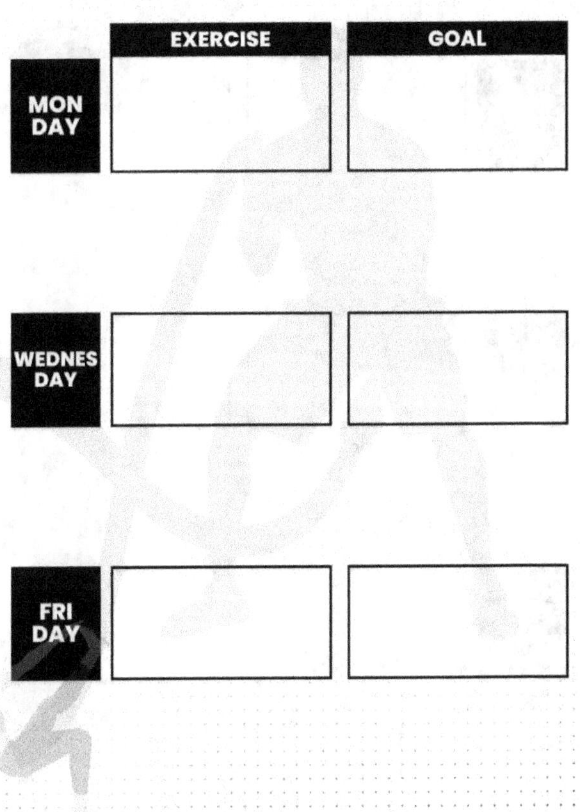

	EXERCISE	GOAL
MON DAY		
WEDNES DAY		
FRI DAY		

WORKOUT PLANNER

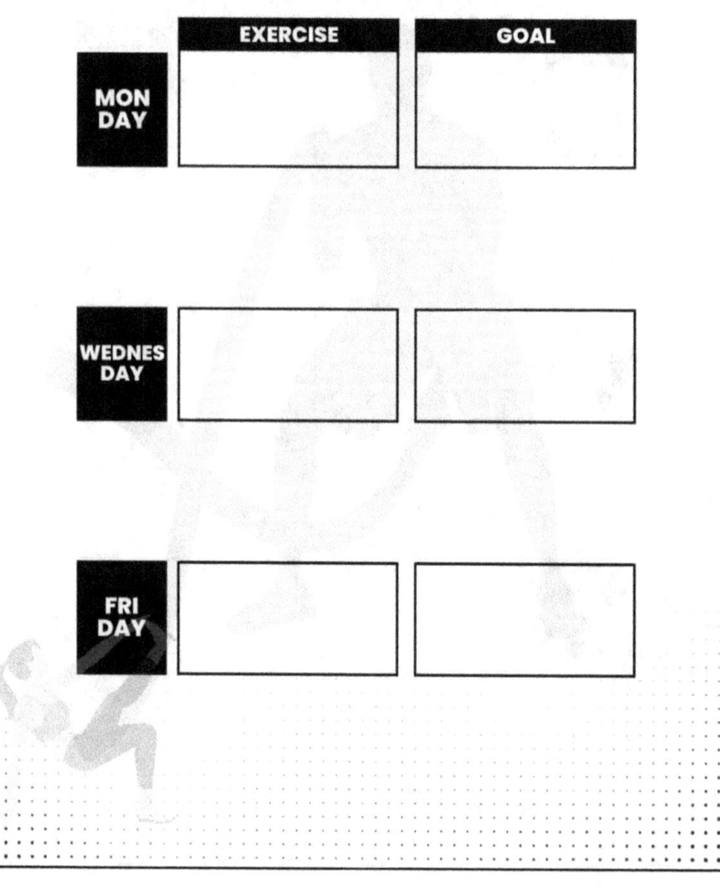

WORKOUT PLANNER

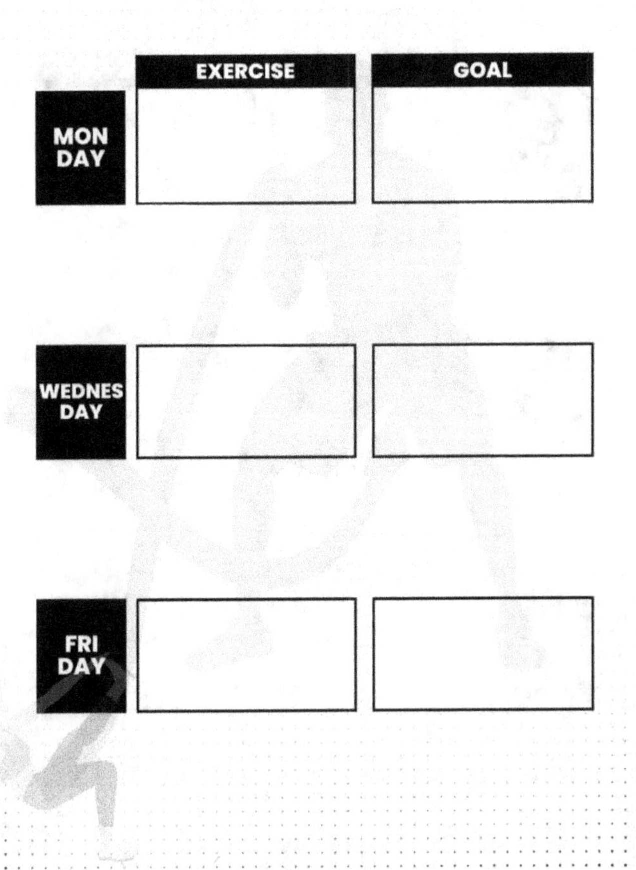

WORKOUT PLANNER

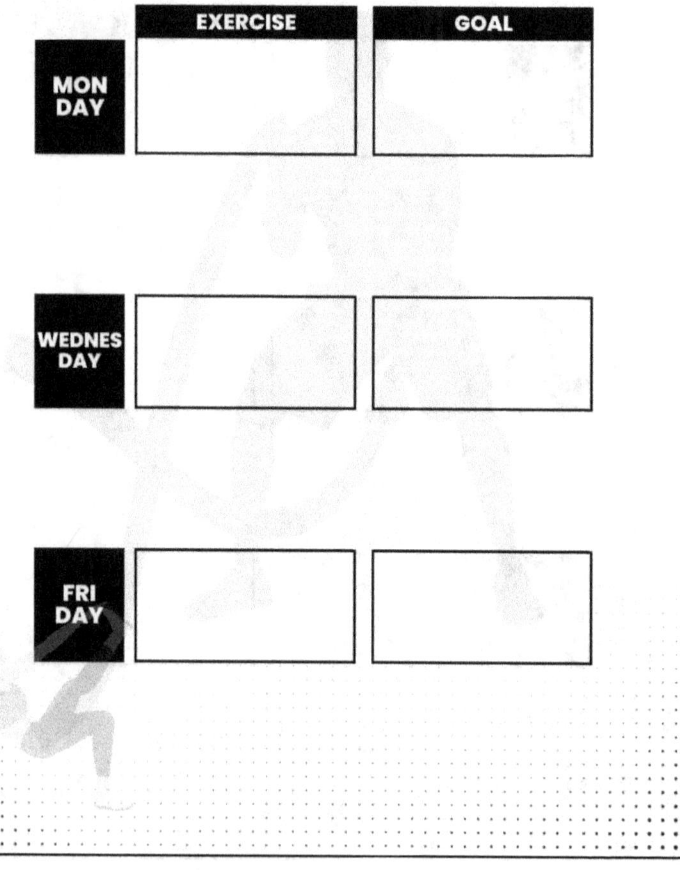

WORKOUT PLANNER

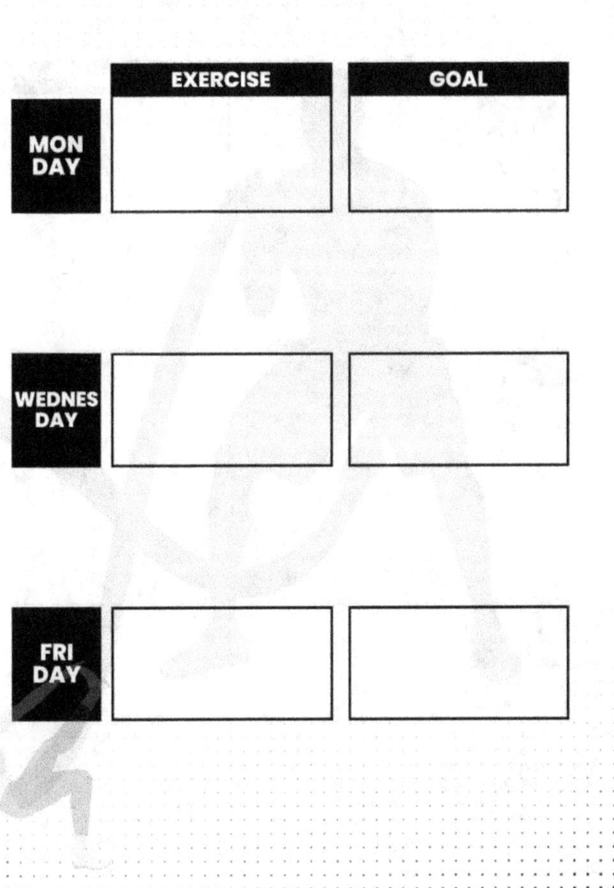

WORKOUT PLANNER

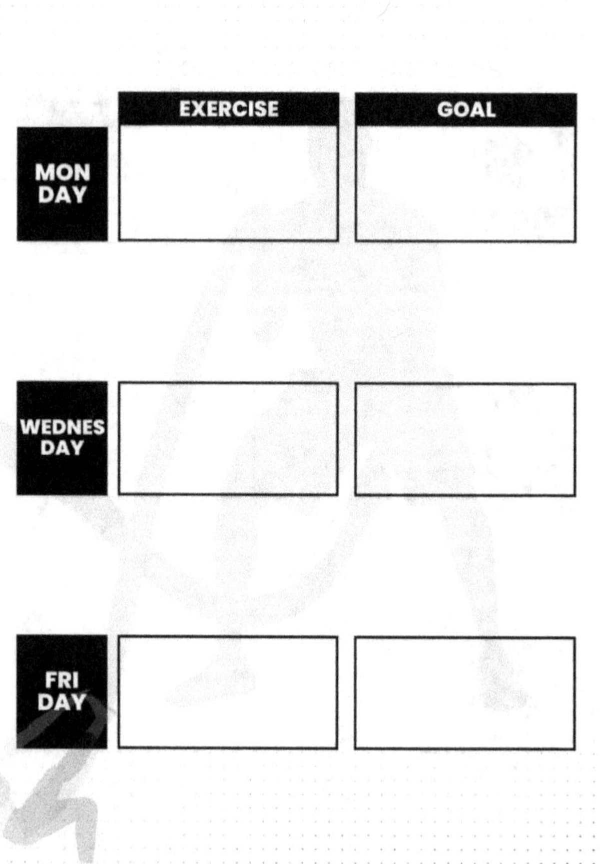

WORKOUT PLANNER

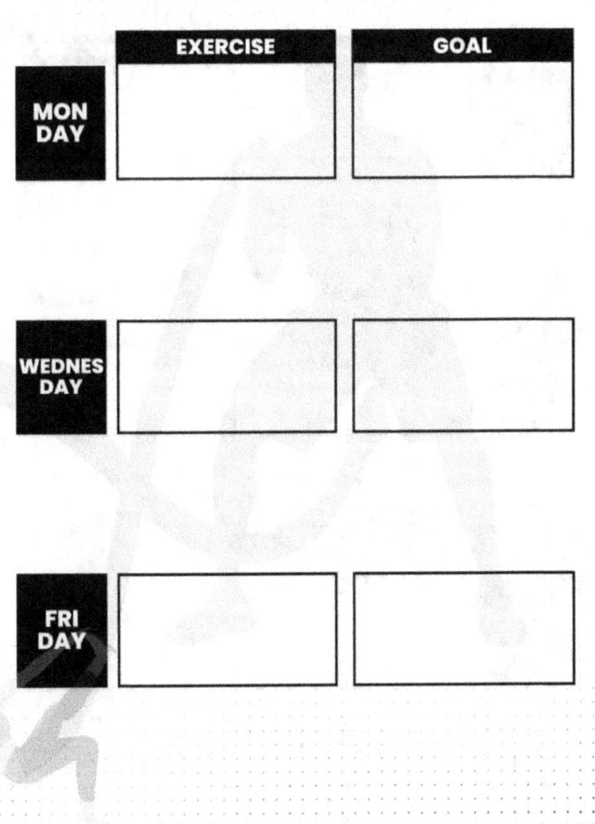

WORKOUT PLANNER

	EXERCISE	GOAL
MON DAY		
WEDNES DAY		
FRI DAY		

WORKOUT PLANNER

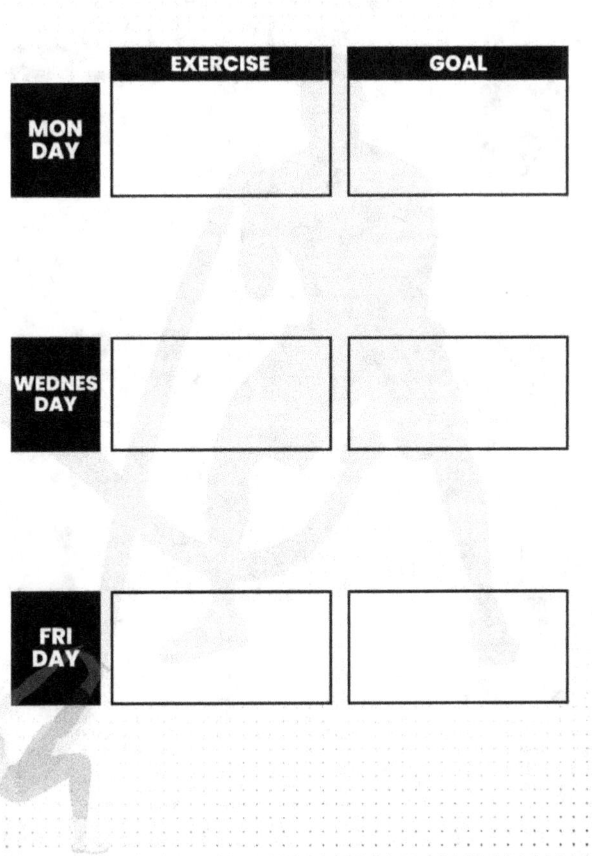

WORKOUT PLANNER

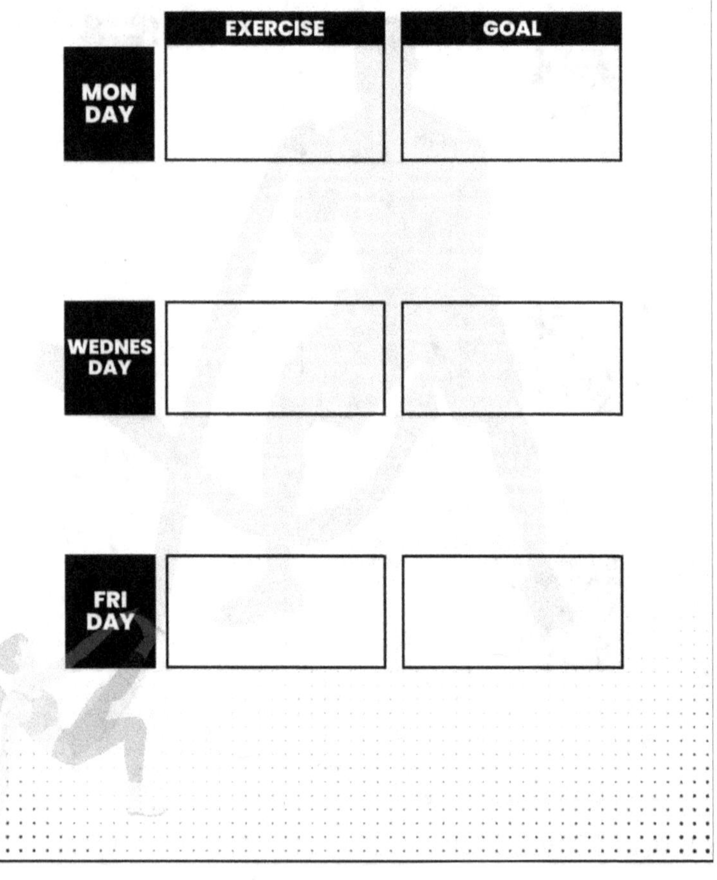

WORKOUT PLANNER

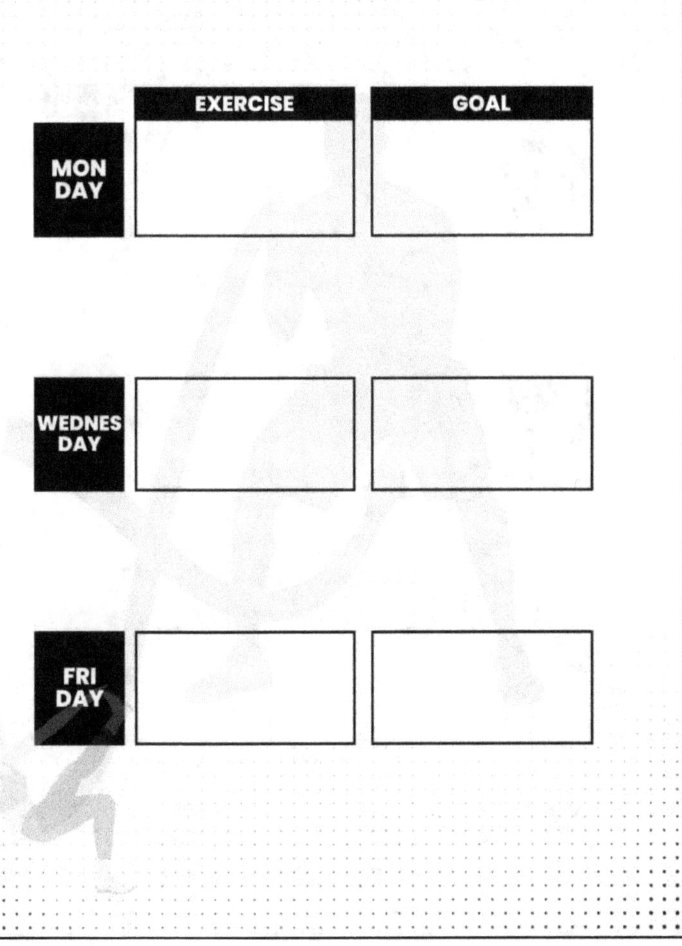

WORKOUT PLANNER

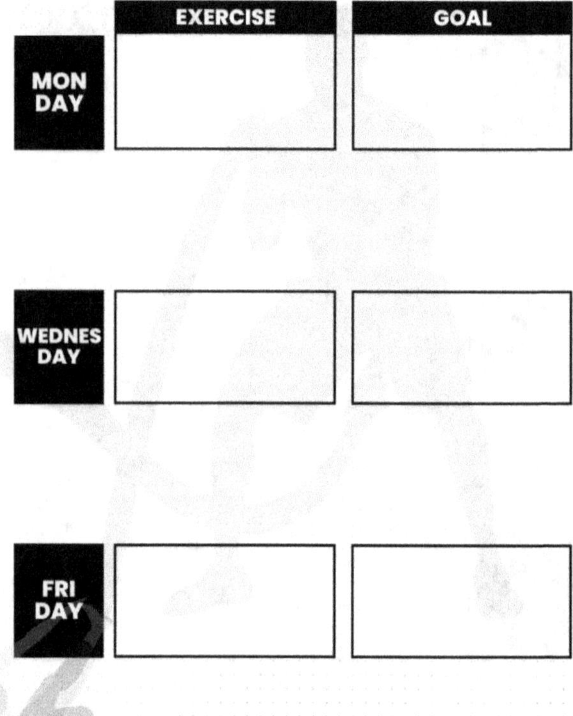

www.ingramcontent.com/pod-product-compliance
Lightning Source LLC
Chambersburg PA
CBHW070948260726
48661CB00003B/1175